# LOST NURSE TO BOSS NURSE

## KANIKA RAJA RN, BSN, CCRN

TINA,

FROM ONE BOSS NURSE TO
ANOTHER, HOPE THIS BOOK
WARMS YOUR NURSING
HEART ♡ ALL THE BEST,

Kanika Raja

# Thank You!

When I wrote my book I had a goal to reach and connect with as many nurses as possible. The more I thought about it, I realized I wanted its impact to be slightly greater. Here is where you come in…

10% of the net proceeds of this book will go to Feeding America and Direct Relief (to be split equally among both). Feeding America's mission is to end the fight against hunger in the U.S. Direct Relief is an international humanitarian aid organization, with a mission to improve the health and lives of people affected by poverty or emergencies. Both charities are well reputed and are known for having high fundraising efficiency ratings.

The brilliant thing about this fundraising effort is the fact that we get to do it together. Each person who buys a copy of this book will have contributed to these wonderful organizations.

Lastly, I would love to hear from you! Connect with me on my website kanikaraja.com. On my website, I have a couple of free gifts that will help in your "boss" nurse quest. This book is my baby. I actually fed and burped her daily. Man, babies are a lot of work. If you would take a moment to leave me a review on Amazon when you are finished with the book, it would mean the world to me. Happy reading ya'll.

*Yes Please!!!*

# Preface

I am writing this preface on April 1st, 2020. As we all know, April 1st is April Fools Day. I have always thought of April Fools Day not so much as a day of practical jokes and pranks, but as a day to celebrate laughter and merriment. If you know me (and if you are reading this book, you will know me pretty darn well by the end), you know that laughter is pretty much my favorite thing. There is no greater euphoria than the feeling of laughing so hard that you can't catch your breath.

I enjoy this day so much that as a kid I always wished for my birthday to be April 1st. My birthday is on December 31st, which entails a celebration of its own kind. In nursing school, I came to a wonderfully weird realization. While taking obstetrics and gynecology, I realized that approximately nine months before December 31st is April 1st. So although I wasn't born on April Fools Day, I may have been conceived on the day! It's quite possible that some version of me was brought into this world on my favorite day. The joke's been on my parents ever since.

It does occur to me that I am discussing the topic of my conception less than several hundred words into my book. It is slightly unusual for you to know me on such an intimate level already. Not many authors would talk about their conception right out of the gate, but most authors are not me. I think it's fantastic for us to have established this strange bond right from the start. Some of the best relationships are forged in awkwardness, and I am happy for us to start off this way as well.

I love April Fools Day, but I must say April 1st, 2020, has not been one of my favorites. The state of the world is quite unfunny right now. Our current situation feels like a chapter from a dystopian novel. COVID-19 has the world in its clutches, and this virus is affecting every one of us.

Nurses care for patients who have been infected by this virus at a more intimate level than anyone. Even though I am a nurse, I am still in awe of all my fellow nurses and healthcare workers. The intelligence and skill you possess are incredible, but your courage is what truly inspires me.

For those of you in nursing school, your clinicals have likely been paused for the time being. Don't be discouraged. The fire inside you to care for others may flicker at this time, but ultimately it will burn brighter than ever. Rest up. Recharge. Keep learning.

I am hoping and praying those not in healthcare are also doing their part to slow the spread of the virus. Be vocal to your friends, family, and community about best practices to minimize the loss of life at this terrible time. I hope and pray that healthcare providers have the resources to continue to perform our job safely. However, hoping and praying may not be enough. If you do not have the proper protective equipment, please speak up to managers and administrators. We have to be loud and unified in our fight to also protect ourselves.

I have no idea how this COVID-19 chapter ends, and that is truly frightening. As I write these words, I can feel myself becoming emotional. It's not a result of fear or frustration, but love for my fellow man. We humans can be such a stupid and self-destructive bunch. However, our overwhelming capacity for good keeps driving me as it will drive many of you. By the time these words are in front of your eyes, I hope that we are on the downhill slope of the pandemic. Despite its challenges, I am so proud to be a nurse. Now more than ever.

To all my fellow nurses (and soon to be nurses), nurture yourselves fiercely and lovingly. Don't forget to care for yourself in your pursuit to care for others.

You are amazing.

See you on the other side of the pandemic real soon. I'll be easy to recognize. I'm the big-haired brown girl with the big smile. I'll be laughing while trying to make you laugh too.

# Acknowledgments

This part is harder than I thought it would be. It's not difficult because I have no one to thank, but the exact opposite. If I could make this 32 pages long and thank every person who has contributed to my development as a nurse and as a person, I would happily do it. For our purposes, though, I will have to whittle it down. If I forgot you, I am going to squeeze you so hard in apology when I see you.

Thanks to my alma mater, Clemson University, and the wonderful professors in the nursing department. When they started with me, I didn't know what a foley catheter was; when they finished with me, I was something resembling a nurse. When I started at Clemson I had a family friend tell me that I would bleed orange in several years. I promptly responded, "That's a bit dramatic!" Ten years later, I stand corrected. If I so much as see someone wearing a Clemson shirt my heart drums with pride. Luckily I haven't needed much phlebotomy work in my life, but I am sure that every blood sample I give is tinged with orange.

To all the incredible nurses and healthcare providers I have had the pleasure of working with, y'all have a twisted sense of humor which, let's face it, keeps us all sane. Thanks to those of you I entrusted with my baby book first. Thank you for taking the time to read it and offer me invaluable feedback.

To my Clemson gang, I love each and every one of you. I met my little tribe when I was in nursing school. You may never guess it now, but my confidence was struggling hard when I met y'all. The anxiety and fear that I felt in nursing school was largely alleviated by the fact that you came into my life at the precise time I needed you the most. I always wanted brothers and sisters, and the universe said "Give me about 20 years and I will give you about 10 of them." Who is cutting onions in here?!

To my corona girls, the period of being a nurse during the COVID-19 pandemic could have been an emotionally draining one. Y'all kept my cup filled (emotionally and otherwise) during this bizarre and potentially isolating time.

Bindu Poudel, you fed my stomach and my soul when I was in nursing school. Any bad*ssery that exists in me is all because of you.

Erica Okwazi, Jenifer Queen, and Bakari Hassan, the three of you have always made me feel like the version of myself that I most want to be. I hope I do the same for you. Vaishnavi Koli, your grace amazes me and I am so happy our paths crossed.

Kruti Patel, you are an incredible person who inspires me every day.

Last and certainly most, I want to thank my Boss and Pops, traditionally known as Mom and Dad. Every bit of goodness in me is completely your fault. No achievement will ever be a greater point of pride than being your kid. I will always be one of those weirdos who will be happy when plans get cancelled with friends if it means I can hang out with my two best friends. I hope this book makes you proud. Because I know you so well, I already know it will.

# Contents

# Chapter 1
........................................................
# Welcome to Nursing!

## Nursing Shift: Episode 1

I walked onto my unit, oblivious to what the shift would hold. I was still in my Bambi nurse phase, bright-eyed and innocent. I pranced up to Barbara who would give me report on my patients. If I had a tail, it would have been wagging. She proceeded to give me the medical history of the patient and told me he was withdrawing from alcohol. Barbara appeared bleary eyed and, quite frankly, done. She further explained the patient was restless and couldn't sit still for more than a few minutes. The doctors were aware, and the patient was on the appropriate withdrawal protocol. She urged me to keep the bed alarm on, as the patient's gait was unsteady and he kept getting out of bed. Then she gave report on my other patient.

As she was making her way off the unit, she turned back and gave me another warning. "I would keep my eye on that one, I don't have a good feeling." I am sure I imagined this part, but the warning came as though it was a prophecy. There may have been smoke and ominous music while she was saying this, but who knows for sure? I went into the patient room to do my initial assessment and Mr. X (as he will be referred to) responded appropriately to all my orientation questions. His gait was also steady. The only abnormality I noted was a slight tremor in his hands. My sweet naive self thought, "Well, maybe he is over the worst of it." Ohhhh, I can tell you are a smart bunch; you already know where this is going. The early part of the shift proceeded with no hiccups. Around midnight, the patient's bed alarm went off. I scurried into the room, and he apologized profusely. "I am so sorry, I forgot to press the call bell. I just needed to go to the bathroom and I didn't want to disturb you." I assured him that it was no problem at all. His gait was steady walking to the bathroom, and even the tremor was gone. When he was tucked back into bed, he asked, "Do you think the bed alarm could be turned off? I get up to use the bathroom several times a night and don't want to keep bothering you." Wittle baby nurse Kanika thought, "Sure, it'll probably be okay." The offer was tantalizing, as my other patient needed constant attention and I had been chasing a train all night, which is to say I had not been able to catch up no matter how hard I hustled. Y'all hear that ominous music again, or is it just me? But thankfully I decided nope, better keep the bed alarm on just in case.

About an hour passed and his call light went on again. I went into the room and my face must have given away the stress I was feeling. (Our unit did not have Patient Care Technicians or Nursing Assistants.) He again gently encouraged, "I really do feel fine. I understand if you need to leave the bed alarm on, but I assure you I am okay." Let's press pause for a second. This feels like the scene in a horror movie where everyone watching is screaming, "No girl, don't do it! Don't walk into that dark shed by yourself!" I ask you now, has that stupid chick ever listened?

Nope, she ALWAYS goes in and the killer is ALWAYS waiting for her. I was the chick in the horror movie and yes, I turned the bed alarm off.

Several hours went by and one of my neighboring nurses got an admission. I went in to help her get the patient admitted. Suddenly, a respiratory therapist bolted into the room and shrieked, "Kanika, room 42!" Room 42 was Mr. X's room so I raced there. This is the part where I think I started hallucinating a bit. Mr. X was sitting at my nursing station (which is a desk between my patient rooms that has a computer and phone). He was naked, his IV dangling from his arm, and the telephone in his hand. The IV site was steadily drip, drip, dripping blood. I yelled, "Sir! What are you doing?!" He slooowly swiveled around like a Bond villain during his big reveal. I'm surprised he wasn't stroking a white cat. He calmly asked, "Am I not even allowed to make a phone call?" As soon as I picked my jaw up off the floor, another nurse and I escorted him back to bed. Unfortunately, this next neuro assessment did not go as well. The patient was speaking to people that weren't there and had no clue where he was. Many exhausting interventions later, the next morning arrived. I gave report to the same nurse from the night before. As I described what happened with the Disney sparkle gone from my eyes, she started laughing. She gave me a tight hug and exclaimed, "Welcome to nursing!"

## Nursing Shift: Episode 2

I walked onto my unit, oblivious to what the shift would hold. Are you beginning to sense this is a pattern in nursing? My nursing heart was a little tougher at this point. Not harder, not jaded, just tougher. In report, I was told that my patient had a severely low potassium level and was unable to move his arms or legs. A critically low potassium level can result in twitching, irregular heart rhythms, and even paralysis. (Normal potassium level is approximately 3.6 to 5.2 mmol/L. (This patient's level was approximately 2.0 mmol/L.) Potassium had been replaced both orally and via IV, but the level was hardly rising. Luckily, the patient had not yet exhibited any signs of cardiac abnormality. The doctors were puzzled as to why the levels were not rising, and for my shift I was to continue his electrolyte replacement protocol.

The patient worked at a company that did commercial painting. One theory the doctors had was the paint thinner he used for work might have been causing the low potassium level.

The nurse told me one more thing. The patient had a criminal history and had been to jail. We were not sure of the exact circumstances though. He had been incarcerated more than 10 years ago, but she wanted to make me aware of the history. Upon hearing this, a little light bulb went on in my head and I thought, "Game face on, Kanika." You may understandably be thinking, "But Kanika, isn't that placing a bias on the patient? Nursing is supposed to be judgment-free." I agree that as a nurse you want your care to be as uninfluenced as possible by your personal judgments. However, nurses are human and certain information (no matter how hard you try) will put you on guard.

I walked into the patient's room to perform my initial assessment. He was warm and friendly, and most surprisingly did not appear to be anxious, despite the fact that he had woken up one morning and suddenly couldn't move his arms and legs. If I woke up one day and couldn't move my limbs, there would absolutely be hysterics. The patient (I'll refer to him as Mr. M) was able to speak and swallow normally. I explained to him that I would unfortunately have to perform blood draws several times overnight to keep checking his potassium level. Again, he was exceedingly calm and polite.

Throughout the shift, I was in and out of the room many times, and Mr. M told me more about himself. He did not give me exact details about his past, but told me he had definitely made mistakes. He kept saying how grateful he was to turn his life around. He spoke lovingly about his friends and family. He plainly stated, "I don't know why but this condition isn't really that scary to me. My life has been so dark in the past, that now each day feels like a bonus. I have a lot of good people pulling for me, and believe that I don't need to fear this."

For the first half of the shift, the potassium level did not budge, and neither did his limbs. Around midnight, his call light lit up and when I went in, he flashed a huge grin. He could just barely wiggle the tips of his fingers and toes. He joyously proclaimed, "I think we are making some progress here!" His next potassium level was drawn at 0200 and the level had risen slightly.

Here comes the kicker. By the time I gave report the next morning, his potassium level was 3.4 mmol/L and he was able to walk! A doctor came to the nursing station where I was giving report, and asked, "Where did Mr. M go?" She expanded "I wasn't here yesterday but my colleague told me he was in that room." I smiled and said, "That's him." She replied skeptically, "But Mr. M couldn't move his legs." I announced, "But I cured him!"

Ok, ok, so I didn't cure him, I just drew the right straw that shift. I can tell you one thing, though. I floated out on a cloud that day. Don't let me give you the wrong impression. Nursing isn't often as fuzzy and rainbow-filled as this, but every once in a while, you get just a little bit of nursing glitter dusted on you.

These two stories highlight the fact that nursing is a mind-boggling spectrum. This spectrum ranges from beautifully gratifying to overwhelmingly frustrating. In your nursing career, you will feel feels that you have never felt before. As a fresh face to the nursing arena you may be wondering, "So what is nursing REALLY like?" Nursing is everything that happened in these two stories, and everything in between. I want to welcome you to this always weird and sometimes wonderful world with open arms. You are one of us now. *Gulp!*

# Chapter 2

........................................................

# The Formerly Lost Nurse

At this point you might be thinking, "Well, those stories are fine and dandy lady, but, um… who the heck are you?" And perhaps more importantly, "How are you going to turn me into a boss nurse?"

Allow me to introduce myself and tell you a bit about what qualifies me to help you in your boss nurse quest. My name is Kanika, and I have been a critical care nurse for five years now. I have been a travel nurse for the last three years. I was born in Los Angeles, and raised in South Carolina. I may have traveled far and wide, but a bit of Southern sweet heat remains in every "Y'all" I utter. I have had the unique opportunity to work in all four corners of this country and with almost every kind of patient. One major exception: birthing babies. I saw one birth in nursing school and my brain said, "Kanika out!" The only time I ever plan to witness that again is if the bundle of joy is coming out of me. As a nurse, I would never have the audacity to say I have seen it all, but I have seen a lot.

Becoming a nurse was not the pursuit of a passion. I was not born with an "I was meant to do this" feeling. I did like the idea of being in healthcare, but wasn't sure if it was the appropriate fit for me. The decision to become a nurse came from crossing almost every other career option off the list. I am not an overly analytical person; I tend to act more on instinct. Normally, I tell my heart and my head to play quietly in the corner while my gut and I act like adults and figure out what needs to be done. However, when it came time to choose a career, the panic started to seep in. I implored my gut to tell me what to do. In response, I heard crickets. It was one of the few times in my life my instincts had nothing to say. So I sat down and made lists to figure out the best course of action.

<u>Things I don't want in a career</u>

No sitting at a desk all day
No sitting on a computer all day
No marketing/sales/being responsible for money
No extensive schooling required (at least to begin my career)

<u>Thing I want in a career</u>

I want to help people one-on-one
I want a clock-in/clock-out schedule
I would love to wear comfy clothes
A solid starting salary

Enlisting the help of my parents and basing it on the lists, we arrived at… nursing. I checked in with my good ole trusty gut, and again asked, "Is nursing right for me?" Once again, crickets. I was

LOST NURSE TO BOSS NURSE

unable to gauge if this was the career path I truly wanted. However, I decided to take the plunge and enroll in an accelerated nursing program.

I had the great fortune of hardly ever being inside a hospital before nursing school. I hadn't even visited any friends or family in the hospital before. This was a blessing. However, this meant nursing school was quite an eye-popping experience for me. I will never forget the day I learned that foley catheters are tubes that are inserted into a patient's bladder. My exact words were, "I insert that where?!" I quickly learned that in healthcare we will stick a tube into pretty much any orifice in the body. Sometimes we create even more orifices to insert even more tubes into.

Nursing school passed in a blur. The thought of all the information being hurtled at me in a span of 16 months still makes me dizzy. However, I earned good grades in nursing school, and miraculously got the first job I applied for. So in essence, all was going to plan perfectly.

My first job was at a Level I trauma facility and I was working in the Medical Surgical ICU. Here is precisely where I started to lose the reins, and the bronco started bucking. Ironically, the fact that I am qualified to get you from LOST nurse to BOSS nurse is precisely because I was THE LOST NURSE.

## I. WAS. LOST.

I want to clarify what I mean by lost. My orientation period lasted for three months, and at the end of it I felt semi-confident in my ability to take on my own patients. However, my first year passed in an anxiety tornado. I didn't know how to take the hundred details being thrown at me and process them. I constantly wanted a more experienced nurse to place her hand on my head and bless any action I was about to take. I was so embarrassed to admit how inadequate I felt. I would sit in my car before every shift and wonder if I had made a giant mistake by choosing this career. I would look up inspirational quotes on my phone and watch videos of puppies being cute, so basically any puppy video. I tried to soothe my fears and tell myself that, in time, this feeling would pass.

Luckily, this story has a happy ending, as the strangling feeling did pass. It took almost a year but that chokehold that I had placed myself in slowly loosened. Looking back on that time now I can fully understand where I went wrong. I did the exact opposite of what I should have done. When anything negative happened or I made a mistake, I extracted the feeling but not the knowledge. I should have extracted the knowledge and flushed the feelings of embarrassment and inadequacy down the toilet.

As you embark on your nursing career, don't make the same mistake I made. If your first year of nursing leaves you feeling defeated, focus on all that you have learned rather than all the times you have failed. Take it from this formerly lost nurse, almost every boss nurse has felt lost at some point in their career. For the rest of this book all my energy will be focused on getting you a one-way express ticket on the boss nurse track. Let's do this!

# Chapter 3

## The Fast Track

Looking back on my first year as a nurse I have come to realize two things.

1. Nursing has a ridiculously steep learning curve. We are talking about Mount Everest-level stuff, folks. Almost all nurses would agree that their first year as a bedside nurse is the hardest. An immense component of nursing is refining the way you approach problems and training your brain to process information effectively. If that isn't enough, nursing is one of the few careers that will challenge you mentally, physically and emotionally.
2. The most successful nurse isn't the one that knows the most facts, or runs around the most. The most successful nurse is the one that prioritizes best and realizes that she (or he) isn't alone.

Over my five years, my little (I mean huge) nursing brain keeps refining the process of delivering solid care without compromising my sanity. Or maybe somewhere along the way I actually lost my sanity, but we'll assume that is not the case. There is no way for me to completely soften your nursing curve. Believe me; if I could, I would turn the curve into a plushy meadow for you. Actually, maybe I wouldn't. How else would you toughen that nursing skin? However, my acquired knowledge and experience can give you a little rocket boost. I will put you on the fast track to boss nurse.

Boss nurses are detail-oriented, but recognize which details are important. We sometimes make mistakes, but we learn from them, and we move on. We understand that there is a difference between working hard and working smart. And our seesaw leans toward working smart. We recognize that sometimes we may have to fight our instincts to roll our eyes so hard that they permanently get stuck backwards. We learn not to be scared to ask for help, and also to shower help on others like Oprah at a Christmas giveaway. We also understand that care isn't always about limbs and lab values. We care for people at their most vulnerable, and our compassion changes lives.

This book can be thought of as a general guideline. You do not have to commit to every suggestion presented. Use your judgement and adapt the suggestions to best suit your nursing style. You are obviously a competent, intelligent person. I mean, you bought my book, so that is a given. Either that or your Aunt Sheila bought this for you as a graduation present. Geez Aunt Sheila, an Amazon or Starbucks gift card would have been just fine! Whatever route this book took to you, I am thrilled that it has.

I was scared sh*tless at certain moments as a new nurse. Although scared sh*tless may not be an appropriate term, I was still full of a lot of sh*t when I started my nursing career. I have taken the tangled mass of yarn that nursing felt like to me, untangled it and presented it back to you. I don't want to fill your brain with false reassurances, but with practical tools to whip out when needed.

Think of me as your fairy godmother. I may not be able to turn your pumpkin into a carriage, but gosh darn it, I will turn you into a boss of the nursing ball! (All without a wand.)

# Chapter 4

## A Chapter on Procrastination

Eh, I'll finish this chapter later.

# Chapter 5

## Bills: How to Get the Job and Actually Pay Them

Remember the nursing glitter that I was talking about earlier? Some nurses get a little extra "excellent memory" glitter sprinkled on them, and some nurses get a little extra "time management." Which glitter was I bestowed with? The "getting the job" glitter.

I have been fortunate in my nursing career to have gotten every job I have interviewed for. I have not gotten every job I *applied* to, but have gotten every job I have *interviewed* for. I'll admit, a component of that is probably pure luck. However, I do interview well. Either that or the nursing angel tripped and spilled the whole bottle of "interview" glitter on me. Again, I want to emphasize that you can do EVERYTHING right and still struggle to find that first nursing job. However, here are the steps I believe will help you in that tricky endeavor of landing a job.

1) Get Comfortable Networking

Networking is more essential in today's job market than ever before. I'll admit, I was wary that networking was all fake enthusiasm and pleasantries. I had to realize that building solid relationships is the foundation of becoming a successful nurse. Talk with your professors and preceptors about more than school. If nothing else, they often have dope stories! Go to career fairs, conferences, call your best friend's aunt who is a nurse and ask her for guidance. Once you establish a connection, it doesn't end there. Continue to foster the relationship. Am I suggesting you become besties with every professional you come across? Heck no. However, investing in people will often lead to beautiful outcomes. Oh man, does this apply to life as well? Hang on, we are onto something deep, people.

## BOSS TIP: Thank Yous and Paying It Forward

Anytime anyone invests time in your success, be sure to let them know how much you appreciate it. A good old-fashioned note is a marvel. But a simple email can also suffice. Somewhere down the road, once you have become a boss nurse and are contributing to cutting-edge research, don't forget what it felt like to be a new grad. Pay forward all that good juju you received. The brilliant thing about good juju is it's limitless, so there is more than enough to go around. (My inner hippie is beginning to show.)

What is priority number one for a new grad? To get a job! Ten points to Gryffindor if you got that correct. Although, I am a #Hufflepuff at heart. But what happens after you get a job? You want to continue to learn and expand your horizons. In general, nurses tend not to be a "kick back and coast" group of people. Many of us are doers and pushers who crave both personal and positional advancement in nursing. The best way to better yourself is to interact with people who are heading down the same professional path as you, but are a few miles ahead. Only a fellow nurse can understand the chaos you will face on a daily basis. If nothing else, you will need to gain your own web of nurses to "vent" with. Vent/Ventilator, y'all I crack myself up.

2) Get an internship/externship/volunteer

I took the accelerated route to obtain my BSN in nursing. My original degree was a BSN in biology, as I had planned to go into healthcare but couldn't really figure out the best path for me. I decided that nursing was the best fit as it was the most flexible. Unfortunately, an accelerated nursing program is somewhat like driving a car with a brick on the accelerator. There is not much time allotted to peeing, let alone an externship. Some of the students in the traditional nursing route were able to secure externships during the summer between junior and senior year. Many of those externships turned into job offers once they graduated.

Inquire with your nursing instructors about any opportunities that they are aware of. Also, contact hospitals directly about any externships/internships. Even if the experience does not directly turn into a job offer, you will have built both valuable experience and connections to help you in the job pursuit. Another option is volunteering. Inquire about any volunteer opportunities at local hospitals/clinics/nursing homes. Remember, (almost) any experience is good experience.

3) When and Where do I apply?

I went to a nursing career fair approximately three months before graduation. I asked every recruiter when was the best time to apply to their hospital and what I could do to set myself apart.

The lady who represented the hospital I was most interested in told me two things. She told me the ideal time to apply was four weeks before I graduate and that my cover letter was important. She said that they had many qualified applicants in terms of grades. She said, "Tell me what makes you unique from every other applicant." I followed both pieces of advice and I graduated with a job in hand.

Now my lovely readers, I hear a few groans from your ranks. You might be thinking, "But Kanika, I have a sterling GPA, have taken every bit of advice, drank the lucky tea my shaman gave me, and donated my kidney. I deserve a job, dammit, and I still don't have one!" I hear you and all my fingers are crossed for you. In essence, each job opportunity you pursue is another dart thrown at a dart board. The more darts you throw, the greater the chance that one will stick. If your first job happens to be your dream one, more power to you! If not, remember this: EVERY job will develop your skills. To cast an even wider net, be open to the possibility of working outside the hospital. There are many opportunities in home health, clinics, nursing homes, etc. You can also opt for receiving alerts on a job search engine. Set a filter for the types of positions you are interested in and be among the first to know when one is posted!

## Where do I apply?

Apply to all the positions that make you most excited first, but then keep going until you get a bite. Do NOT stress about the fact that your first job isn't exactly what you wanted. Even a PRN position can get your foot in the door.

## When do I apply?

Apply two to three months before graduation. Contact the hospitals (or whichever facility you are interested in) and ask them the ideal time to apply and any other recommendations they may have. In my case, the ideal window was four weeks before. It is amazing how often employers will tell you specifically what you need to do to get the job. All you have to do is take the initiative to ask and then follow through.

4) The Application
  The DOs and DO-NOTs

## *DOs*

DO: Mention if you have a BSN right off the bat. Many hospitals are seeking magnet status, and including the BSN after your name carries a lot of weight.

DO: Trim the fat off your resume. Nursing managers are not likely to be interested that you worked at TCBY for three summers. (Did y'all know that TCBY stands for The Country's Best Yogurt? #TheMoreYouKnow.) Sometimes we fall into the trap of padding the resumé, but avoid that temptation. Keep it clean and concise. Try to keep all your experience related to healthcare, even if it is not paid experience. Your whole resume should fit onto one page.

DO: Include any nursing clubs/committees you are a part of, particularly if you held any leadership positions.

DO: Ensure that the job description meets the experience you have. I wouldn't waste much time applying to a job that specifically states "two years experience required." The buzzword that should set off beautiful bells in your head is "experience preferred." The rarer gems are positions tailored to new grads (such as nursing residencies). Apply away to those!

## DO NOTs

DO NOT: Send an incomplete application. For example, if the application requires you to attach your BLS and ACLS certification, be sure to do so.

DO NOT: Slap a generic cover letter on every application. When you are slogging through several applications a day, changing the cover letter can feel exhausting. However, if you are applying to a position, your cover letter should reflect why you want a job in that specific unit. Generally, you may only have to modify a sentence or two for different positions. Take the time to do it.

A funny or interesting anecdote on the cover letter can often set you apart. Not surprisingly, this is my bread and butter. No one else is quite like you. If you can convey that and how it will make you a great nurse, mention it.

DO NOT: Send anything with any misspelligs or badder grammor. (*wink.) They will glare like bulbous zits.

DO NOT: Use funky fonts, headings, or colors. This is no time to break out the Copperplate Gothic Light. Stick to a nice old-fashioned Times New Roman or Arial. Keep the resumé as visually clean and streamlined as possible.

5) The Interview

There have been certain moments in life where my idiosyncrasies have paid off. I (gasp) sort of enjoy going to the dentist, standardized tests, and yes, interviews. I hear y'all thinking, "Ok, we are dealing with a straight-up sadist here." Hang with me, my friends. For some reason, the wiring in my brain prevents me from fearing interviews. I don't really understand it; I just consider it a happy mechanical failure and go about my business. If the thought of an interview makes your palms sweat and your right eye twitch, allow me to help.

The best way to reduce your fear is to flip your perspective. Don't view an interview as a big bad beast who is trying to expose your flaws. It is simply an opportunity. Think of the interview as a conversation. You are not on trial, no need to act like you are. Let's break it down...

### Pre-Interview

1. Ensure you know where to go on the day of the interview. Your anxiety will balloon if you are running around on the day of the interview trying to find the correct meeting place. Go to the site before the interview to make sure you know where to report and where to park.

2. I feel that certain clothes affect my attitude. Most of us have that certain dress/shirt/accessory that puts us in boss mode. Wear an outfit that is professional, comfortable, and makes you feel confident. Try it on the night before to ensure there are no missing buttons, tiny holes, stains, etc. Look polished. Keep nails short and clean, perfume/cologne to a minimum, and have a hairstyle that does not cover your eyes or face. This should go without saying, but not too much cleavage, ladies. Again this should go without saying, but not too much cleavage, gentlemen.

### BOSS TIP:

Have an extra layer. Wear a shirt/dress/blouse but have a nice cardigan/jacket/blazer to throw on top if needed. My own body language can get a little squirmy when I am either too hot or too cold. This tip helps to ensure a little extra comfort.

3. Prepare a little portfolio (folder) that includes your resumé, cover letter, certifications, references, etc. Plan to leave the portfolio with your interviewer. You might choose to include a little "About me" page that highlights just a few things about you, for example, the fact that you speak another language, you like to hike, or you have a German shepherd who is the light of your life. Keep it sweet and short. This tip isn't imperative, but I believe this humanizes you and keeps you from becoming another face in the interview crowd.

4. Do an activity the day or evening before that relaxes you, particularly before your first interview. That might be a yoga class, a pedicure, a massage, or some nice takeout. Guys, I am looking at you, too. Don't tell me that hot stone massage isn't calling your name. This step might feel a little indulgent (especially on a tight budget) but trust me, feeling relaxed translates to feeling confident.

## Sample Questions

Certain questions are tailor-made for nursing interviews. I don't recommend memorizing an answer to all questions, but having some familiarity with potential questions can be helpful. I suggest knowing a bit about the facility as well. Learn the mission statement, any specific goals, and recent advancements. Have a solid scroll through the facility website to learn this information.

Remember, personal examples are generally better than generic answers. Again, you might be asked questions you did not expect, but your preparation will help you improvise as needed. Have a friend or family member ask you these questions so you can have a general idea of how you would like to answer. Better yet, grab another nursing buddy and practice together. The aim is not to dazzle the interviewer but to come across as competent, positive, and personable. I have provided answers to two questions to get the ball rolling. All other questions have little tips to keep you on the right track. Ensure that your answers fit you!

*1) Tell me about yourself/Why did you become a nurse?*
If the "Nursing Interview" was a play, these would likely be the opening lines. No need to restate your entire resumé. This is your chance to set the tone for the interview, and lay the groundwork for the questions to follow. Also, any background you provide should generally tie into nursing. This is not the time for "I enjoy long strolls on the beach and smooth jazz."

My response:
I am excited to begin my career and put my degree in action. I knew I wanted to go into healthcare, as I have a passion for service. The challenge and flexibility of nursing made it the best fit for me. Ironically, my fear of hospitals as a patient is exactly why I went into nursing. Something in me said that if the hospital is where I feel most vulnerable, I want to be a professional that makes it less scary for others.

I think the light-bulb moment for me happened when I was 10 years old. I had an awful fall while rollerblading and had to get 17 stitches below my knee. I was bawling as my parents took me to the doctor. After the nurse and doctor convinced me that they weren't going to amputate my leg, I calmed down slightly. Their constant warmth and reassurance zapped all my fear. I think the seed of caring for others was planted that day.

I feel confident that my strong academic background has set me up well to take on this position. I know I have a lot to learn, and will work hard to do so.

*2) Why do you want to work at this facility?*
Your response should highlight the vision and goals of the facility. Include how they are compatible with your approach as a nurse.

*3) Are you a team player?*
The short answer: yes. Highlight an example where you demonstrated good teamwork. There is no problem with honesty. If there are certain times when you prefer to think or work as an individual, it is perfectly acceptable. However, working effectively as a team member is essential to nursing.

*4) Describe a time you had to deal with a difficult situation/Tell me about a time you were placed in an ethical dilemma.*
Your answer should be geared toward resolution and what you learned from the experience. Patient safety should always be the highest priority, and your actions should reflect that. If you felt you could have handled the situation better, explain what you might change in the future.

*5) Tell me about your greatest strength as a nurse.*
Of course we all have our own particular strengths, and your answer should reflect yours. Some wonderful attributes for a nurse to have include being hardworking, a team player, compassionate, intelligent, flexible, an effective multi-tasker, etc. Your answer will likely include one or more of these qualities.

*6) Tell me about your weaknesses/what you find most challenging about nursing.*
Ummm, my greatest weakness is that I am a little too amazing. Yeah, no.

I always find this question a little tricky. On one hand you want to show that you can recognize areas of improvement in yourself, but you don't want to shoot yourself in the foot, either.

My response:
My weakness is that I can get intimidated by strong personalities. I have trouble speaking up when I feel the person I am working with doesn't respect my opinion. I understand that there will be times when I will need to be assertive, especially if it affects patient care. I know that this feeling can be quite common as a new nurse. I think the key is that confidence will come with experience. (I might elaborate a little more in an actual interview, but that is the gist.)

*7) Do you have any questions for us?*
YES! By having a couple of well thought-out questions, it will show that you are genuinely interested in the position and convey confidence. Remember how I said that an interview is a conversation? If the interviewer wants to make sure you are a good fit, then it's reasonable for you to understand if the position is a good fit.

Ask questions that you truly want to know the answer to, no need for fillers. However, stray away from questions regarding pay and time off. Your interviewer's interest may go from red hot to ice cold if you carry on about the moolah.

## Potential Questions to Ask
- Could you tell me more about the orientation process?
- What are the expectations for new grads/new nurses?
- What are the short-term and long-term goals of the unit?
- What advancement/educational opportunities do the nurses have?

- Could you tell me more about nurse-to-patient ratios and the typical patient population?

## During the Interview

Get there early. Keep it simple. Smile. Breathe.

## BOSS TIPS:

- Talk as though you are speaking to a favorite professor. Essentially, speak respectfully but without intimidation.
- Keep a small bottle of water with you. If nerves make your mouth dry, the water is right there.

## Follow Up

Whew! The interview is over and hopefully it went swimmingly. Reach out to the nursing manager (or whoever interviewed you) after the interview. The crème de la crème of the follow-up is a handwritten note. If not a note, send an email or have a quick phone call in which you thank them for the opportunity to interview. End by saying you look forward to hearing from them. Don't underestimate the value of following up. This is one last chance to leave a positive impression. One note, phone call, or email is enough; we don't want to roam into stalker territory.

If you do not get the position, ask the interviewer or manager if there is anything you could have done differently or better. Honestly, they will probably tell you that there was just a strong pool of candidates and you narrowly missed out. However, occasionally they might give you useful feedback that you can apply to your next interview.

If you receive the first job, fantastic! If not, no problem. You now know what to expect for the second interview. Lather, rinse, and repeat until the position is yours. Chin up, a job is headed your way.

## Confession- A Note on the Dream Job

I am one of the chosen ones. I wanted to work in an ICU when I graduated and bam! I got the ICU job! However, looking back, I wonder if that was the best place for me to start. I often wonder if starting on a step down or telemetry unit might have been better for me. Or perhaps no matter where I would have started, the first year would have been just as difficult. One of my friends started in the same Medical ICU as me, and after one year her literal response was "Nope." She transferred to Neonatal ICU and was far happier. I think I have harped on this point enough but let me just one last time reiterate that your first nursing job is exactly that: your first nursing job. If you happen to love it and stay until retirement, great! If not, soak up every ounce of knowledge you can until the next step on your path.

# Chapter 6

## Orientation: How to Squeeze All the Juice Out

### Prior to Orientation

You have gotten your first job! Whoot whoot… what now?

Do a little more research about the hospital, specifically your unit. If possible, have a brief chat with your unit educator/manager. Find out more about the typical patient population and any other information they recommend you know prior to your orientation. Even if they say that you don't need to learn any additional information, this gesture shows you are highly motivated to learn. Drive to the hospital at the time of your shift to get an idea of the traffic and approximate time to get there. (I love ya, GPS, but we both know you are not always on point.) Make sure you know where you are expected to park and if badge access is needed. With security's blessing, walk around the campus/hospital, learn which floors house which units. Learn where radiology, CT, MRI, lab, blood bank, and any other area specific to your role, are located.

LOST NURSE TO BOSS NURSE

Learning all this prior to orientation may feel like overkill, but honestly, familiarity with the hospital layout can really help save time later on.

## 1st Day of Unit Orientation

GET THERE EARLY. Nothing will give you more anxiety or lead to a worse impression than showing up late on your first day. Get up a little early, take your time getting ready. Savor that double-shot latte. If you have to wait several minutes because you are early, so be it.

There are several nursing supplies that I recommend you have day 1. This list should apply to most nursing units in a hospital setting. You can supplement this list as you progress and decide what additional items are useful to your practice. Also, let me take a moment to plug an underutilized gem: fanny packs! Yup, you heard me, fanny packs. No longer a relic that only rotund fathers use on vacation, they are a boss nurse's best-kept secret. Truly, it is wonderful to tote your own little supply cabinet right around your waist. Remember, together we can make it cool!

Basic Supply Checklist
- Nursing watch
- Stethoscope
- Clipboard
- Retractable pens
- Pen light
- Nursing scissors
- Black permanent marker
- Optional: small notepad

## BOSS TIP:

Have the essentials on you whenever possible. These include nursing scissors, black permanent marker, tape, alcohol swabs, flushes, and your stethoscope. Let's say your preceptor is in the middle of showing you how to do a dressing change and realizes he forgot his scissors at his station. Nothing will make you look like a boss as much as whipping out a pair of scissors.

### During Orientation

Orientation for a new graduate typically lasts between three to six months depending on the specific unit, sometimes even less. This is your time to learn and try as much as you can before you are on your own. Speak up about wanting to do as many types of procedures as possible in that time. I cannot emphasize enough that watching a procedure is not the equivalent of performing a procedure. When you feel confident that you know the steps of a procedure, ask your preceptor to observe/assist while you perform. Anytime there is a complex or less common procedure happening on the unit (and your patients do not require any immediate care), ask your preceptor if you can go observe. The beauty of this is your preceptor will see you are highly motivated to learn and will usually begin to offer up additional opportunities as well. You can also request for the charge nurse to make you and your preceptor aware of any such procedures on the unit.

## BOSS TIP:

Be vocal (though polite) about anything you feel you need that you are not getting from your orientation.

## Head-to-Toe Initial Assessment

Your initial assessment may not be one of the more juicy aspects of nursing, but it is the holy grail of patient care. Since I will be a broken record on the importance of the initial assessment, I am going to provide a checklist of the most common and essential elements. You want to quickly cover all the body systems, but have a problem-focused approach. For example, if the patient has come to your unit post bilateral knee replacement, you probably won't do an in-depth neuro exam (unless indicated due to patient history or an acute change). Know what the expected findings would be for the patient based on their history and diagnosis. Let's break down a general head-to-toe assessment. Again, based on your unit and specific patient, the assessment might vary.

## Basic Assessment Checklist (Including Common Equipment)

1. Wash your hands and introduce yourself to the patient
2. Check their identification band
3. General status
   1. Does the patient appear to be in any distress or have any critical concerns?
   2. Is there any abnormality that needs to be addressed immediately?
4. Vital signs
   - Heart rate, blood pressure, oxygen saturation, respiratory rate, and temperature
   - Pain level
5. Neurological
   - Facial symmetry (note any facial abnormality)
   - Orientation status/ability to follow commands

- Visual acuity
- PERRLA (Pupils Equal/Round/Reactive to Light/ Accommodating)
- Strength and coordination of extremities
- In critically ill patients, you may also be assessing for a cough and gag reflex

6. Cardiovascular
   - If the patient is on telemetry, analyze rhythm
   - Auscultate for S1 and S2. Note any abnormalities such as murmurs, rubs, etc.
   - Peripheral pulses (brachial, pedal, etc.). Note equality and strength of pulses
   - Edema — location and severity of pitting (if pitting edema is noted)
   - If the patient has invasive hemodynamic monitoring (arterial line, central venous pressure, etc.), then you will also assess those lines and values
   - Capillary refill
   - Temperature of extremities. Look for any abnormalities that suggest compromised circulation

7. Respiratory
   - Rhythm and depth of breaths. Look for any signs of shortness of breath
   - Auscultate lung sounds. Note abnormalities such as crackles, wheezing, etc.
   - Note if the patient is on supplemental oxygen (ventilator, nasal cannula, etc.). If the patient is on a ventilator, you will also want to record ventilator settings (tidal volume, respiratory rate, Peak Expiratory End Pressure (PEEP), and oxygen level). Note the size of the endotracheal tube (ETT) and the location of the tube

- Assess for cough and secretions
- Chest tube — check output, site, dressing, and wall suction setting if applicable

8. Gastrointestinal
    - Assess the mouth. Note sores, loose/missing teeth, etc.
    - Auscultate bowel sounds in all four quadrants of abdomen. Palpate the abdomen and note distension, pain, or masses
    - Note time of last bowel movement, and bowel movement quality/color. Check if the patient has a rectal tube and record quality and quantity of output
    - Assess nutrition status and know patient's diet orders
    - Nasogastric (NG), orogastric (OG), or other feeding/suction tube present? Note depth in cm.
        1. Used for feeding/suction/clamped?
        2. Quality and amount of secretions if applicable
        3. Tube feed type and rate if applicable
        4. Tube feed residuals? Also confirm feeding tube placement per unit policy. Initial confirmation will most likely be via x-ray, and thereafter will be auscultation for an air bubble

9. Genitourinary
    - Urine output—color, quality (sediment/clots/odor) and quantity
    - Assess foley, suprapubic, or condom catheter if applicable
    - If the patient is on dialysis, examine the access (arteriovenous fistula, ash cath, etc.)

10. Musculoskeletal
    - Will vary greatly based on patient condition and diagnosis but will include test for generalized muscular strength and range of motion

- The assessment for the musculoskeletal system can often be incorporated into the neuro exam since you will already be asking the patient to follow commands, lift extremities, etc.

11. Integumentary/lines/equipment
   - I like to combine all three of these together. When I assess the patient's skin for any breakdown/irregularity, I also examine any lines and equipment the patient has.
   - Skin — assess temperature, moisture, turgor, wounds, dressings, pressure sores, etc.
   - Lines — assess for color, skin condition around the insertion site, dressings, and ensure all lines are untangled. Check for patency and blood return (if appropriate). Make sure you know what medication or fluid is infusing in each line. This is also a great time to ensure any drip rates and pump settings are accurate.
   - Equipment — check Sequential Compression Devices (SCDs), sleeves, braces, casts, etc. If not already done, make sure all monitors have parameters appropriate to the patient. You will also want zero/re-calibrate any hemodynamic lines.

## BOSS TIPS:

- Ensure no equipment is pressing continuously against the patient's skin and causing breakdown. One of my patients had a sat probe on his ear. It had not been rotated for several shifts and his ear developed a pretty gnarly sore.
- I mention this again but try to do report at the bedside. It is amazing what can get missed when we don't actually have the patient in front of us when we give or get report.

LOST NURSE TO BOSS NURSE

- Don't be hard on yourself; the initial assessment is a slippery little sucker. It seems easy at face value, but it can be tricky to remember all the components. But never fear, your fairy godmother is here! I love a good mnemonic and here are two that can help you remember the steps of an assessment.

**IIV**
**I**ntroduce
**I**D
**V**itals

**N**ursing **C**an **R**eally **G/G**et **M**e **S**tressed, **L**et's **E**at! (**NCRGMS-LE**)
**N**euro
**C**ardio
**R**espiratory
**G**I/**G**U
**M**usculoskeletal
**S**kin
**L**ines
**E**quipment

Because let's be real, the best way I deal with stress is by eating. Hangry, table for one? Side note: 90% of the time in nursing, when you find yourself feeling cranky you are either thirsty, hungry or you need to pee. Amazingly, at times it's all three. At the same time.

## Calling the Doc

Get comfortable calling doctors as soon as possible. I can almost guarantee that the first time you call a doctor you will feel like you botched it. The first couple rounds of awkwardness will dissolve and you will soon become a pro. Here's how it's done...

## Calling MD Checklist

1. Your name/your unit/patient name/patient room number/ what patient is admitted for
2. Relevant background information (i.e. vitals, labs, history)
3. Explain specifically what the problem is, often you will have a suggested intervention ready
4. If the doctor places a telephone order, be sure to repeat back the order to ensure accuracy

Always have the patient's electronic chart open for unanticipated information the doctor might ask. When you don't have the chart open, inevitably the doctor will throw you a curveball that you were not expecting. Also inevitably, if the computer chart is not open, every computer will decide to load at the pace of a patient who just had hip replacement surgery.

## SBAR—Situation/Background/Assessment/Recommendation

This acronym was probably drilled into you in nursing school. It is one of the golden nuggets of nursing. Using this as a framework for calling an MD is often helpful.

I am going to give you a quick sample conversation to demonstrate how the outline should work. We will assume that the MD that you are calling is the attending for the patient.

Nurse: Hi Dr. Sands. My name is Kanika and I am calling from unit 4H. I am calling to report a lab value on Sue Taylor in room 19. Her hemoglobin was 7.4 g/dl at 1600. There is a note in the chart to notify a MD when the hemoglobin is below 7.5

g/dl. Her hemoglobin prior to this lab draw was 7.7 g/dl and was drawn on September 17th at 0400. She was admitted for an acute GI bleed on September 15th. She received 2 units of PRBC on the 15th. I do not see any new bleeding at this time.

Doctor: Are Ms. Taylor's vital signs stable at this time?

Nurse: Yes. HR is 86, O2 sat is 98% on room air, BP=127/72. No other abnormalities noted. She also has another hemoglobin and hematocrit lab ordered for the 18th at 0400. Do you want to transfuse at this time or place any other orders?

Doctor: No, let's wait and see the results of her next H and H (hemoglobin and hematocrit). Let us know if you see any active bleeding or if she becomes symptomatic.

Nurse: Ok, I will monitor for any signs of bleeding and ask the night shift nurse to monitor as well. Thank you.

Drop the mic and walk away like a boss.

## Boss Level Skills

1. Make sure you are calling the appropriate MD for the problem. For example, a patient may have a cardiologist, pulmonologist, and a surgeon on board. If the patient starts having an irregular heart rhythm, call the cardiologist. In a rush you may accidentally call a doctor that is not the right fit for the issue. However, still let the primary physician know if a consulted MD places an order for a procedure, scan, etc.

2. Ask your nursing neighbors if they also need to talk to the MD you are calling before you call. By no means am I saying walk around the whole unit like, "I got Dr. Sands on the line, does anyone need anything?" However, asking a couple of the nurses around you can help avoid multi-

KANIKA RAJA RN, BSN, CCRN

ple calls to the same doctor. This tip especially applies on night shift if the doctor has to be paged at home. Again, nursing is all about judgement. This tip goes out the window if you are calling the MD for an urgent matter and don't have time to ask other nurses.

## Documentation

Warning. The following is a nursing truth bomb. You can be the most hardworking, knowledgeable, and competent nurse in the world but until you document appropriately, it ain't worth much. In my version of paradise, documentation wouldn't be necessary. Alas, we don't live in that world, and appropriate documentation is vital.

You may be familiar with the nursing mantra, "If you didn't document it, you didn't do it." There are two major reasons why proper documentation is important. First, the information you provide will lead to effective patient care. Second, poor documentation can potentially make you and your facility vulnerable to liability. The clearer your documentation, the clearer the picture will be for the entire healthcare team. Keep in mind, thorough documentation doesn't necessarily mean lengthy. Convey all the necessary information without writing an epic saga. Most electronic charting symptoms will have blank areas that you simply have to fill in. However, here is one sample of a nursing documentation note, only to illustrate how your mental approach should be if a note is ever required.

Here are examples of two nurses documenting pain medication given:

1. Gave pain medication ordered for strong pain in the left shoulder. Rechecked pain level after 30 min. Pt. states, "It feels much better."

2. Gave 650 mg acetaminophen for pain in the left shoulder. Pt. verbalizes soreness in left shoulder, non-radiating. 5/10 on numeric scale. 2/10 pain at 30 min recheck after administration of medication.

Both examples convey that the patient was having pain in the left shoulder and that the medication given provided relief. However, the second example tells you the medication, the dose, and a rating for the severity of the pain.

You may be thinking, "Well, duh Kanika, no good nurse would chart like the first example." However, you would be surprised at how sloppy charting can get when you are rushed and tired.

## Between you and me

At my first nursing job, I worked with a wonderful nurse that we'll call Mary. Mary was a compassionate, sharp nurse who provided quality care to her patients. She had emigrated from another country and English was not her first language. Her charting was more of a stream of consciousness than straight facts. I remember one day that she gave me report on one of her patients. The patient was withdrawing from alcohol and it was apparent that he may not have had a shower in several days. I was reading through her notes for the shift and one note said, "Patient did not smell good, so I gave him a bath. I asked the family to also bring in some nail clippers, because they are too long." Did your eyes pop open? I'm pretty sure mine did when I read it. This story is not intended to make fun of Mary or the patient, but to highlight that subjective charting, (which includes your thoughts, emotions, and opinions), should be avoided. Make your charting as objective as possible. If a patient's statement is pertinent to their care, then include "Patient states..." in your nursing note.

KANIKA RAJA RN, BSN, CCRN

Chart as you go. It is absolutely soul-sucking to get to the end of a horrible shift and realize you haven't charted much. Also, the details of what happened several hours ago can become foggy. At the very least, jot down any time medications were given or any important interventions were done. Sometimes you may not be able to avoid getting delayed in charting, but try to get the initial assessment charted ASAP. This will also help establish a baseline in the event your patient's condition deteriorates during the shift. This is something that I struggled with early in my nursing career, but I found that if I could at least get my initial assessments charted early, it took a lot of pressure off the rest of the shift.

## Legal tip:

Be cautious about charting ahead. At 0750, you may be tempted to chart that your patient was resting comfortably at 0800; after all, it's only 10 min away. However, let's say your patient falls out of bed at 0755 (I hope this never happens to you!). If your charting reflects that your patient was resting at 0800 when there is a chart review, you may open yourself up to liability.

## Nursing Report

Nursing report is the opening and closing curtain of the shift. You will definitely develop your own style of giving and getting report.

Here is the information you will include (at a minimum):

- Patient information (name, age, allergies)
- Diagnosis
- Code status
- Relevant history
- Isolation precautions
- Mobility status

- Doctors on board and any other teams consulted such as wound care, palliative, etc.
- Head-to-toe body systems assessment. The level of detail you go into for each body system will be dictated by the patient's diagnosis
- Significant lab results (complete blood count, electrolytes, etc.)
- IV and other line locations (central line, arterial line, etc.)
- Restraints
- Fluids and medications currently infusing
- Significant events of last shift
- Plan for oncoming (your) shift

(On my website, kanikaraja.com, I have provided a sample report sheet for you.) Give and get report at the bedside. This is becoming standard practice in many hospitals. This especially applies when the patient is new to you. Initially when management started pushing bedside report, I felt like it wouldn't really make a big difference in care. I stand corrected.

Here are some of the benefits of bedside report:

1. Puts patients at ease when they know what the plan of care is and who will take over care
2. Can reduce medication errors by ensuring pump settings and drip rates are accurate
3. Can visually examine skin for:
   - wounds
   - dressings
   - pressure ulcers
   - IV INFILTRATIONS

I can't tell you how many times I forget to tell the oncoming nurse something, but upon seeing the patient my memory would be jogged.

## BOSS TIP:

I tend not to let things get under my skin, but we all have our breaking point. I am looking at you, report interrupters! Constant interruptions disrupt the train of thought. Once that train is derailed at the end of a 12-hour shift, it is hard to get back on track. It is frustrating to be describing a patient's respiratory status and the oncoming nurse asks, "But when did she have her last bowel movement?" My face be like: [insert exasperated expression of your choice].

But you are better than that! Let the nurse get through the report and then ask any remaining questions you have.

### Between you and me

I'm not going to lie, nursing is a juicy career. You will hear and see things that will make "Jerry Springer" seem like wholesome family programming. You will find that during report, some nurses will tell you more about your patient's baby daddy issues than about their ventilator settings. Frankly, it can be quite entertaining. All I would say is, be cautious. Protect the integrity of your patients, and protect your license. To any of you out there asking, "But Kanika, have you ever indulged in some light gossip?" I would respond, "Ooh, unfortunately that's all the time we have on this subject, folks."

# Chapter 7

## I Insert that Where?!
## Tips for Common Procedures

I could cover every aspect of every nursing procedure in depth, but by the time I finished I would be 97, you would be retired, and robots would be doing our jobs anyway. Although as soon as the first bodily fluid hits them, they will short circuit in a cascade of sparks. Yay, job security! You have learned the principles of most common procedures in school and likely practiced on a cold, unflinching rubber dummy. You are now progressing to the world of warm, squirming humans. I can smell your excitement from here!

My **Fast 15** is a list of common procedures for most nursing units. I recommend performing these as often as possible while you are on orientation. If while performing any of these procedures you find yourself tensing up, imagine a mini Kanika on your shoulder cheering you on. I have provided tips of what I would be shouting whilst on your shoulder. I am going to move forward with the assumption you already have familiarity with each procedure I will touch base on. I will focus primarily on the most common nursing interventions and troubleshooting tips.

DISCLAIMER! Each of my tips has been useful to my practice, but your unit/hospital policies and procedures should always override my two cents. Also, each patient is unique. The process for a procedure may change based on their diagnosis or anatomy. I am in no way advocating a "my way or the highway" mentality. As nurses, we all develop our own techniques, and my helpful hints are purely to supplement your knowledge as your own skills develop. I am constantly learning new tips and tricks from nursing colleagues, so the skill refining never ends. In fact, I hope that one day as I am walking down the street, one of you stops me and tells me a sick new technique for starting an IV. I am waiting, y'all!

# The Fast 15

1) Medication Administration

It seems to me that every time I check, there are additional RIGHTS of medication administration. When I was in school, it was five rights and now it has progressed to 12 according to certain sources. By the time my grandkid graduates from nursing school, it will be up to 93 rights, and that is all the nursing school curriculum will have time for. For our purposes, I think the following eight are the most essential.

Remember the eight RIGHTS of medication administration.
1. You have the RIGHT to remain silent… wait whoops, wrong kind of right!

Here we go…
1. RIGHT Patient
2. RIGHT Drug
3. RIGHT Dose

4. RIGHT Route
5. RIGHT Time
6. RIGHT Reason
7. RIGHT Result
8. RIGHT Documentation

The rights appear self-explanatory, and generally they are. The most important piece of advice I can give you regarding med administration is NEVER give a medication if you are unsure what the intended effect is and what side effects to be looking for. ALWAYS take the time to look up the medication prior to administration if you are not comfortable with your knowledge of it. Also, always assess whether the medication had an appropriate effect in an appropriate time frame. For example, if you administer an anti-hypertensive medication, ensure you recheck the patient's blood pressure within the appropriate time frame.

- Only collect one patient's medications at a time and minimize interruptions. I know I have made a point of advising you to cluster care, but this is one of the exceptions. It is surprisingly easy to mix up patient medications. Luckily, most facilities employ electronic scanning to minimize these errors, but best safety practice is still one patient at a time.
- Make a habit of telling the patient what medications they are being given and educating them. This has two benefits. One is that the patient will often help you catch errors. They may tell you they no longer take a medication, that they now take a different dose, etc. Also, at times, medications may be entered in error by providers or pharmacists. Make sure to double check with the patient if possible to avoid giving incorrect meds or incorrect doses. The sec-

ond benefit is the reinforcement of knowledge the patient will receive, particularly if they are going to be discharged with any new medications that you are administering.

## 2) IV insertions

The golden skill of the nursing world. Remember the nursing glitter? Well, the nursing fairies were a little stingy with their "IV" glitter on me. I am not bad at starting IVs, but I have seen some true IV whisperers. There are more tips on IV insertions than there are recipes for grandma's chocolate chip cookies. I am constantly trying to improve my technique at this skill, and the following tips have proven the most helpful.

- Have all your supplies ready prior to insertion of the needle. Have your dressing/tape/flush/catheter all prepped/primed/open so no one-handed maneuvering is required.
- Don't rush! Make sure you truly feel/see an appropriate vein and stabilize the vein as much as possible by holding the skin taut. If the patient is squirmy or jumpy, it may be helpful to have another nurse or patient care tech help you stabilize the arm.
- Ask your patient if they have had an IV before and where it was placed. If it worked before, it may be a solid choice again.
- Be sure to verify the patient doesn't have limitations on which arm can be used. If they have an AV fistula (for dialysis access), or have had a mastectomy on one side, then they may not be able to have an IV placed on that side.
- If it is difficult to palpate a vein, wrap the patient's arm in a warm blanket or towel for several minutes and then try again. The warmth will help vasodilate the veins and often make them plump up. An additional option is to have the

patient dangle their arm for several minutes and let gravity help plump up their veins.

- With difficult sticks, it is often easier to use a blood pressure cuff rather than a tourniquet. The constriction will be more uniform and spread out over a larger surface area. I am a big fan of this tip, and have had a lot of success with it!
- Start with low veins and work your way up. If you start with a higher vein and are unsuccessful, you may lose the option to try lower veins.
- Make sure you insert the right IV for the job! If your patient is on his way to CT, generally at least a #20 gauge in the antecubital (AC) or similar large vein in the forearm will be required. If your patient has an extended infusion to be administered, the AC is a poor choice because the catheter will bend and obstruct flow every time the patient bends their arm. However, if you need something ASAP in a critical situation, the AC can often be a good vein for quick access.
- Once you get a precious IV in place, try not to lose it! Check to see if taping is secure and not pulling on the insertion site. Make sure you flush the IV every several hours to ensure patency. Disconnect tubing if there is no medication/fluid infusing to avoid the IV accidentally being tugged and pulled out.

3) IV infusions

- Check your pumps! Ensure that IV medications are infusing at the correct rate during report.
- Ensure that every medication infusing together is compatible. Most electronic charting systems have a link to

KANIKA RAJA RN, BSN, CCRN

check IV compatibility. As a newer nurse, I once started two IV medications that were infusing through the same line and (rookie mistake) forgot to check their compatibility. Luckily I was still in the patient room when I noticed that the medication was actually crystallizing in the line. Visually it was awesome, but in terms of patient safety, not so much.

- Be on the lookout for infiltrations and extravascular leakage of medication! I have seen (this time not on my patient) an extravascular leak of norepinephrine and it was gnarly. Several days after it was caught, a large portion of the patient's skin around the initial IV site had become necrotic. Don't let it happen to you!

- Many medications (including vasopressors) are ideally infused through a central line due to risk of tissue ischemia if there is an extravascular leak. However, the policy can vary from hospital to hospital.

4) Packed Red Blood Cell (PRBC) administration

Or as I like to call it, the "reverse vampire." For our purposes, I will focus on PRBC administration, as it will generally be given the most often of all the blood products. I have a juicy (both literally and figuratively) story about PRBC administration. This story involves another phrase that student nurses dread... "skills check-off." The horror, the anxiety, the overall sweatiness of skills check-offs is something I will never forget. I mentioned earlier that I have very little test anxiety. However, when it comes to practical demonstrations of my knowledge, my body tenses completely. Even thinking about skills check offs as I am writing this is making my buttocks clench. Real classy imagery, right folks? Evokes feelings of Hemingway or Faulkner.

48

*Let's set the scene.*

All of us nursing students were in a holding room, being called in for our check-offs one at a time. Each person who completed their check-off walked back through the holding room, but we were not supposed to discuss what skill we performed with the students who were still waiting. We were to draw a skill from a hat and perform that for an instructor. Skills included starting an IV medication, inserting a foley catheter, inserting a NG tube and, you guessed it, blood administration. I drew blood administration and felt fairly confident about performing it. My hands were shaking slightly as I removed the cap from the blood bag (which I assume was corn syrup and food coloring, although who knows?). The port where I was to insert the IV spike was a little loose and as I went to insert it, I tipped the bag slightly towards me. This is where I blacked out, because the next thing I realize is that I have "blood" all over my arms and my WHITE — yes, WHITE — scrubs. I wordlessly turned to my instructor and pleaded for mercy with my eyes. Bless this sweet, sweet lady because this is what she said: "We have been using that bag all day, and the insertion port is so loose. That is not your fault, carry on." I somehow was able to demonstrate the rest of the skill appropriately and I passed my check-off.

Here is the best part. When I went back into the holding room, I had a twisted smile on my face and what appeared to be blood all over me. I cannot imagine what was going through the rest of the students' minds as I left the room! My europhia soon passed as I realized that I did not have spare clothes and now had to drive home. If for some reason I had been pulled over by a cop on the way home, I am absolutely certain I would have been a murder suspect. Fortunately, no cops were seen on the way home, and your girl remains jail-free!

Blood Administration Checklist

- The patient will need at least a #20 gauge IV for administration; a #22 gauge is generally not recommended.
- Ensure you have a signed consent and order to administer prior to administration.
- If the patient has a history of reaction, ensure the lab and doctor are aware.
- Vitals will be taken and documented (at the minimum) prior to administration, 15 min after the start of administration, at least every hour thereafter until infusion is complete, and once after administration is complete.
- PRBC administration must be completed in less than four hrs.
- Appropriately document start time, unit #, IV used, and any other pertinent information prior to administration. Most electronic charting systems will have a specific area where blood product administration is documented.
- Some hospitals require a two-nurse check-off, some no longer require two nurses. Be aware of your hospital's policy.

# BOSS TIPS:

- Know the signs of an adverse reaction. These include fever, rash, tachycardia, hypotension, chest pain, and shortness of breath. Essentially if anything looks significantly off from baseline, immediately stop the infusion and make the lab/MD aware!
- Tell the patient (if they are cognitively able) to make you aware if they feel any abnormality during administration.
- Set the pump to have the blood infuse for only 15 min initially. The initial rate will generally be around 75mL/hr.

Check the vitals at this 15 min mark before increasing the rate as appropriate for the patient.

5) Blood draws (labs)

In terms of skill set, performing a blood draw is similar to placing an IV. There are just a few tips to keep in mind.

- Similarly to placing an IV, ask the patient which veins they usually get blood drawn from. During my shift only yesterday, I was looking for a good vein in my patient's right arm. Right before I went to insert the needle, the patient told me, "They usually have a really hard time with the veins in my right arm. Usually the veins in my left arm work way better." I am so glad she spoke up before I stuck her!

- Here is another truth bomb about nursing. Almost all nurses will mislabel a blood sample at some point in their career. I chose a particularly unfortunate time for my mislabeling experience. I had a patient who was having an acute GI bleed. The patient was becoming pale and his blood pressure was beginning to drop. I sent a stat CBC and PTT with my other patient's label on it! When the lab informed me of the mistake, I was so frustrated with myself. Double check that you have the correct label on every sample/specimen you send. Don't add to the mislabeling statistics!

- Try to consolidate sticks as much as possible. Whenever you send a blood sample, ensure you don't need to send another color tube soon. There is nothing worse than walking into a patient room with your tail between your legs because you have to stick them again for another lab that was due 15 min later.

6) Specimen collection
- Once again, check the label. Make sure all information needed is on the label, and that the correct patient label is used.
- Ensure that specimen cups are closed securely. Nobody needs a urine or stool sample to leak in the tube station!

## STORY TIME!

There was a wonderful nurse who I worked with who had been a nurse for at least 40 years. This lady was sharp, sassy, and didn't have much "patience for nonsense," as she called it. I worked with her one night shift when the lab had called her a couple of times for various issues. During the most recent call, they told her that the stool specimen she sent on the patient did not contain a sufficient amount of stool for analysis. "Debbie" got a crazy look in her eyes and sweetly told the lab, "No problem, I will send another one." I knew some sh*t (both literally and figuratively) was about to go down. Debbie filled another specimen cup TO THE BRIM with stool. When I say filled to the brim, I do not exaggerate. There wasn't even space for a fart left in that specimen cup. About 15 minutes later, Debbie called down to the lab and asked, "Do you have enough stool to run the analysis now?" Better put some ice on that burrrrrn, lab!

7) Applying electrodes/12-Lead Electrocardiogram (ECG or EKG)
If any of your patients are ordered to be on telemetry or are in the ICU, they will require constant cardiac monitoring. Generally they will be monitored via five electrodes. Remember, smoke over fire (black over red) and clouds over grass (white on top of green), and dirt (brown) in the middle!

If the patient has a cardiac rhythm change, then the doctor may order a 12-lead EKG. Bear with me a moment. When I first learned about 12-lead EKGs I was so confused. If there were 10 electrodes on the patient's body, then why the heck was it called a "12-lead"? Just in case any of you are still scratching your noggin like I was, a 12-lead essentially means "12 views." Each view shows a different spatial orientation of the heart. My EKG lecture starts and ends there. I highly recommend all of you take a 12-lead EKG class to have a better understanding of the heart's electrical activity and various rhythms.

8) Oxygen Delivery Methods

Ah yes, let's talk about that tiny little detail of patient care: breathing. The SpO2 (oxygen saturation) value is generally maintained above 92% on whichever delivery method is suitable for the patient, but there are exceptions to this. Also, a higher oxygen saturation level isn't always better. Oxygen delivery is a complex matter, with several factors taken into account. For our purposes, I am going to concentrate on the delivery methods I have seen most commonly. I want to refresh your memory on the options available, but generally you will work with a respiratory therapist when any option other than a simple nasal cannula is used.

1. *Nasal cannula*
   Generally utilized when the adult patient requires 4 L/min (or less) of oxygen delivery to maintain an adequate saturation.
2. *High-flow nasal cannula*
   If the patient starts requiring greater than 4 L/min, then they will be on a high-flow nasal cannula. The oxygen is humidified to decrease irritation and inflammation

of the nasal cavity. When utilizing a high-flow system, the flow rate (L/min) and the oxygen concentration (FiO2) can be titrated as required.

3. *Venturi Masks and Non-Rebreathers*

Here is another honesty session between you and me. I rarely see venturi masks or non-rebreather masks being used. In certain conditions, if the objective is to have a higher FiO2 delivery while decreasing $CO_2$ retention, they may be used. Generally however, if the high flow isn't cutting it, the patient is on their way to BiPAP boulevard and if that doesn't do the trick, intubation station is the next stop.

4. *CPAP and BiPAP*

A CPAP (Continuous Positive Airway Pressure) machine is used to help a patient maintain an open airway while sleeping. This machine is generally used by patients to treat sleep apnea. Sometimes patients may use their home CPAP if they are in hospital. Generally, the patient is able to use their own CPAP, or a respiratory therapist can aid them.

A BiPAP (BiLevel Positive Airway Pressure) machine functions similarly to a CPAP. However, the pressure of the air supplied during inhalation is greater than the pressure of air during exhalation. With a CPAP machine, the pressure of air during inhalation and exhalation remains constant. BiPAP machines are used on patients who are having breathing difficulty due to conditions such as COPD, pneumonia, and respiratory distress. The BiPAP is generally the next option after high-flow nasal cannula because it can supply both oxygen and the pressure to deliver the oxygen to the lungs. However, if the patient is having trouble maintaining consciousness or there is a risk they can't protect their airway, intubation may become necessary.

5. *Bag Valve Masks*

BVMs (or you might hear them referred to as ambu bags) are most commonly used during CPR or if the patient is in the process of being intubated. BVMs provide both ventilation (move the air into the patient's lungs) and adequate oxygenation. The proper use of BVMS is taught during both Basic Life Support (BLS) and Advanced Cardiac Life Support (ACLS) training. Most units will require nurses to have BLS certification and critical care nurses will need to obtain ACLS certification.

6. *Endotracheal Tube (ETT)*

This is the most invasive form of oxygen delivery. An ETT is inserted into the patient's trachea and connected to a ventilator. Various settings can be manipulated on the ventilator in response to the patient's condition. Again, I won't go into detail about ventilator settings, but just know that several parameters on the ventilator can be adjusted to meet the patient's ventilation and oxygenation needs. Remember that a chest x-ray will need to be obtained after intubation to confirm proper placement of the tube.

## Incentive Spirometry

If I had a dollar for every time I walked into a patient's room and they were blowing into their incentive spirometer instead of sucking air in, I would be sipping mai tais on an island somewhere! An IS is often used for patients after surgery, extubation, or if they have respiratory issues. Encourage your patients to use the IS if they are ordered to. It truly does help patients strengthen their lungs, increase their lung capacity, and reduce the chances of pneumonia. Don't let them get lazy with their IS.

9) Bladder scans/foley catheter insertions

When I graduated nursing school, foley catheter insertions felt like a yellow belt in karate. If I could just master this skill, I would be one step closer to becoming a nursing sensei. In case this skill makes you apprehensive, allow my former anxiety to put you at ease.

*Flashback to my first Med-Surg clinical.*

I was attempting my first foley catheter insertion. The patient was a medically obese female and had a yeast infection. Yup, that's right. My instructor was standing at the bedside and talking to the patient's daughter. I was nervous, and from the second I opened the sterile package, everything went a bit hazy. I put on the sterile gloves and started to clean around the meatus, and then froze. I had not opened the lube package or put the syringe on the inflation port! I just kept looking from the catheter to the patient's meatus and back again like a ping pong match from hell. My already large eyes became saucers and I silently pleaded for my instructor's help. Luckily he turned around and wordlessly opened a new package of sterile gloves (which he had kept in his pocket) and lubed the tip of the catheter and inserted the syringe on the port. Hallelujah!

He debriefed me after, and told me I would try another insertion next week at clinical. My second foley insertion was on a middle-aged gentleman and it was a wham bam, thank you ma'am operation. If any of you are wondering if that means it went well, it went perfectly. As you know, gentlemen provide a much clearer target (not to say their catheter insertions are always smooth sailing either, since there can be anatomical challenges there too).

# BOSS TIPS:

- On the ladies, the smaller hole on top is the urethra, the bigger hole on the bottom is the vagina. If the catheter is accidentally inserted into the vagina, it can be kept there to avoid the same mistake with the next kit.

- Locate the urethra before you break open the sterile package, particularly if the urethra will be difficult to locate. Trust me, you will know which patients will make it difficult to locate. And if you're not sure, find it first.
- If you are left handed, stand on the left side of the patient. If you are right handed, stand on the patient's right side. Once you touch the patient with your sterile glove, that hand CANNOT touch sterile objects.
- Prepare the items in the sterile package before you clean the urethral meatus.
  1. Open the betadine swabs OR pour the betadine on the cotton balls
  2. Attach the sterile water syringe on the inflation port of the balloon
  3. Lube the tip of the catheter
- For your female patients (who are in no respiratory distress), having the bed in a slight reverse Trendelenberg can help facilitate an easier insertion.
- For removal — once all the water is removed from the balloon, have the patient take a big breath in. As they exhale, pull out the catheter. I find patients report less discomfort using this method. It may be that forced inhalation and exhalation distracts them.
- If the patient hasn't voided in several hours, ask the patient if they need to void. Most units have a policy set in place for the patient to void no longer than six hours after a foley catheter is removed. Some patients have to be coaxed to void. It is amazing how often the patient will suddenly be able to pee if they think there is a possibility the catheter

may need to go back in! I had an elderly gentleman tell me recently he was going to squeeze until something came out because he wasn't getting the terrible "peeing snake tube" again! Lo and behold, he was able to void!

• A bladder scan machine can always be utilized to see if the patient is retaining. Patients who are post-surgery can often have trouble with retention, so bladder scan if needed. We don't want anything to burst down there.

10) NasoGastric (NG) tube insertion and tube feedings

Nursing is such a strange game. As I mentioned before, pretty much any orifice on a patient's body can have a tube inserted. Of all of the tubes we insert, the NG tube insertion is the one I hate putting patients through the most. I have a strong gag reflex, so to put a tube into someone's nose and down their throat is almost as awful for me as it is for them. However, NG tubes are the best way for patients to receive nutrition and medication if they are unable to swallow and eat normally, or to drain gastric contents if needed.

## TIPS

• Measure from the tip of the nose to the ear, then to the xiphoid process. (The xiphoid what?! The xiphoid process is located roughly in the center of the chest, just below the sternum.) Go ahead and mark how deep you plan to insert the tube based on this measurement with a piece of tape, especially if you are a beginner.

• If the tube coils into the patient's mouth, sometimes placing the tube in ice water can help firm up the tube and make it easier to go down. Be sure to check your unit's policy on this.

- If the patient is alert and oriented, encourage them to take several deep breaths beforehand and then just focus on swallowing. Once the tip is past the nasal cavity, it's time for them to swallow, swallow, swallow.
- Auscultate for an air bubble once the tube is in, and ensure the tube is well secured to avoid it slipping out. The only thing worse than inserting an NG tube is reinserting an NG tube.
- Check your unit's policy for obtaining a chest x-ray to confirm placement. If the NG tube has a guidewire, leave the wire in place until after the x-ray. Once the position is confirmed, make sure to remove the guide wire.
- If the patient is on tube feeding, make sure you check residuals. If the patient is not digesting the feeding appropriately, tube feeds may need to be stopped to avoid aspiration. Each unit has a protocol for residual limits, so be sure to follow those.

11) Chest tube care

Of the more common pieces of equipment that nurses use on a day-to-day basis, chest tubes intimidate me the most. They are not overly complex once you gain familiarity with them, but it took some time for me to feel comfortable with them.

Most Common Nursing Interventions for Chest Tube Setup and Maintenance

- You will gather supplies and assist at the bedside for chest tube insertion. You will also generally fill the water seal chamber with the appropriate amount of sterile water (generally provided with the chest tube kit). You will set the wall suction based on the doctor's orders.

- You will monitor and record the quality (color, presence of clots, etc.) and quantity of the output hourly. Generally, doctors will want to be notified if the chest tube output is greater than a certain amount per hour, for example if the output is greater than 100mL/hr.
- Tidaling (a gentle oscillation up and down) will be seen in the water seal chamber as the patient breathes. If there is no tidaling, it could indicate a pneumothorax or that the patient's lung has re-inflated. In either case, make the doctor aware. Also, if there is constant bubbling in the water seal chamber, it could indicate an air leak. You will need to determine the source of the leak and intervene as appropriate. Often an air leak indicates a problem with the chest tube system connections. Make sure all connections are secured.
- If a patient's chest tube comes out of the patient accidentally, you will apply an occlusive dressing to the site and tape it on three sites. Leave one side untaped to prevent a pneumothorax.
- The supplies you will want to have on hand include: petroleum gauze, 4 inch x 4 inch sized dry gauze, tape, two clamps without teeth, and sterile water. Ask your preceptor to demonstrate how to set up a chest tube, what to do if the system is compromised, or the tube becomes dislodged.
- If you need to attach a new chest tube collection system, then put the tube attached to the system in one inch of sterile water to maintain a water seal.

12) Skin/wound care

I will not cover wound care in depth, but want to emphasize a couple of important aspects:

- The initial assessment of your patient when they are admitted is essential. Make sure you document any wounds, skin abnormalities, ostomies, surgical incisions, etc. on your initial assessment. Continue to reassess the skin per your unit's policy and/or doctor's order. Some units have a policy to take pictures of wounds to be placed in the patient's electronic chart. If the patient has wounds that are not appropriately documented initially, the assumption will be that the wound was developed in hospital. It is in the best interest of the medical staff, the hospital, and the patient to know when any skin abnormality first occurred.

- Check the buttocks and back! Sores and wounds are most likely to be missed in the areas that are least visible so make sure the sacral area, perineum, back, any skin folds, heels, etc. are examined carefully.

- Always keep this in the back of your mind. As nurses we want to try our best to not send the patient out with any new problems. Prevention of the problem is the name of the game! Skin can break down easily, and as nurses we have to try to minimize damage, especially for those patients who are unable to move.

- Turn your patients per your unit's policy and access their circulation.

- Keep pressure points protected. Elevate heels and elbows on pillows. Some patients may even require medical boots that keep their heels protected.

- Make sure no equipment or lines are pressing into the patient's skin. Rotate oxygen saturation probes, blood pressure cuffs, and any other equipment per your nursing discretion to minimize harm.

- If the patient has wounds that need to be cleansed/dressed, follow the orders in regard to supplies to be used and frequency of dressing changes. Some surgeons want to be the ones to take off the initial dressing after surgery, so check with them prior to any dressing removal or cleansing intervention. If you change the dressing, mark with the date, time, and your initials to keep track of when the dressing was last changed.

13) Physical Restraints

The unfortunate reality of our job is that, at times, restraints will be required for the patient's own safety. Intubated patients may require restraints to prevent them from accidentally removing the tube prematurely. However, no medical condition automatically warrants the use of restraints.

Restraints should only be used if other alternatives are exhausted. Nurses will have to gauge if the patient is truly a harm to themselves or others prior to placing restraints.

General guidelines for restraints:
- Make sure you have an order for restraint and ensure the order matches the restraints applied. The order should also include how long the restraints can be applied for. The most common order is bilateral soft wrist/upper extremity restraints.
- Before placing the restraints, explain to the patient why they are being placed. Even if you think the patient doesn't understand you, it is your duty to explain to the patient that the restraint is only being placed for safety. If the patient has designated someone as a contact person, make them aware that restraints have been placed.

- Make sure the restraint is applied properly. When in doubt if it has been placed properly, check with another nurse who is familiar with the restraint.
- Most units will require nurses to assess and document on restraints every two hours. Be sure to truly check whether the restraints are secure and not compromising the patient's circulation. Sometimes, patients will pull at restraints and make them tighter or looser, so be on the lookout.
- Again, between you and me, restraints can be a hot spot of liability. Be sure you are protecting both your license and the patient by assessing and documenting appropriately.

14) Transports

Most hospitals will have a transport team for patients, however sometimes they don't cover the whole 24 hours. Also, ICU and other high acuity patients require a nurse during transport. I want to give you a checklist of what to be mindful of during patient transport as the nurse. I don't have many phobias, bring on the bugs/heights/scary movies and I yawn in their faces. However, I am slightly claustrophobic. (None of y'all ever use that against me, ok?!) One of my fears is being stuck in an elevator alone with a patient. Even as I am typing this, I feel my heart rate accelerating. Also, if the patient is on a ventilator, a respiratory therapist has to come with me, so whew!

Transport Team Transfers (The nurse will not accompany and these will be non-critical patients)
- Most units will require the patient to have a "Ticket to Ride." The ticket can be used for room transfers or if the patient is going for a scan/procedure such as a CT. This ticket will include any pertinent information about patient's

code status, allergies, mobility, IVs, oxygen requirements, etc. Try to have the ticket to ride ready prior to the arrival of transport to avoid hastily filling it out at the last second. Also, being prepared will keep the transport team from getting behind.

- If the patient is on oxygen, let transport know to bring a portable oxygen tank. Make sure the tank is full (or at least close to full) prior to transport. Also per most policies, if the patient is on 6L of oxygen/min or greater, generally the nurse will have to accompany them.

- If the patient is ordered to be on telemetry, ensure they are placed on the appropriate telemetry box or portable monitor. Make sure the battery is charged and will not die during transport.

- If the patient has fluids infusing, they can generally be stopped during transport to avoid compromising the line. I like to saline-lock my lines during transport if it is okay for the patient's maintenance fluids (ie. normal saline, lactated ringers, etc.) to be stopped for a short time. However, certain infusions/fluids should not be stopped. Check with the charge nurse or provider if you are unsure.

- Make sure your patient is appropriately covered during transport. Keep them warm and keep their "parts" tucked out of sight. Sometimes we get in a go, go, go mode and forget to protect the patient's dignity.

Additional Consideration for Critical Patients
- As I mentioned before, these patients will require a nurse during transport. Make sure the appropriate equipment is on the patient to monitor vitals during transport.

- If your patient is on a ventilator, a respiratory therapist will set up a portable ventilator. Also ensure that you travel with a bag valve mask (ambu bag) in case of emergency.

## BOSS TIP:

Give the RT a heads up if you anticipate traveling for a procedure. Trust me, you want the RT to be your friend, and they will not be too friendly toward you if you constantly tell them you need to go to CT right now versus you need to go to CT in 30 minutes. (I think I hear the faint sounds of RTs cheering in the distance.)

15) Bed Baths and POOP!

I have been tip-toeing around an unpleasant topic until now. Take a deep breath and then hold it in, my friends. Let's talk about POOP! Unfortunately, 60% of your stress in nursing will be related to patients not having bowel movements, and then choosing to have a bowel movement at the most inconvenient time. The longer I am a nurse, I realize how essential "plumbing" is to the well-being of a patient. If they are stopped up, it leads to a whole cascade of problems, and if they are not, then we are dealing with another type of cascade entirely. Ok Kanika, time to chill with the bathroom innuendo.

Always assess a patient's bowel sounds carefully, and if their bowel sounds are diminished, then ensure it is an expected finding. For example, post-surgery patients may have slowed bowel sounds. Also, if the patient is on any narcotics, they can also slow the passing of bowels and lead to constipation. If the patient is having trouble in this regard, make sure they are on the appropriate stool softeners and laxatives or obtain an order for them.

One of the most important things to remember is how embarrassing it can be for the patient to use a bedpan or a bedside commode. Reassure them that it is not a big deal and put them at ease as much as possible. Any one of us can imagine how uncomfortable it must be to try to have a bowel movement without the privacy of a bathroom, so always try to keep that in mind.

Now we are about to really delve in. I am going to give you my tips on how to clean a patient who has had a bowel movement in bed or simply needs a bed bath. If any of you are squirming right now, let me assure you that, soon enough, cleaning a patient will become second nature and you'll practically be able to do it blindfolded. Have I mentioned that nursing is a weird career?

- A mask with either vaporub or essential oil applied to the inside can help to deal with the aroma associated with the task. Some might say wearing a mask is embarrassing for the patient, but I think it is ok, especially if you are particularly sensitive to aromas.
- Obtain wipes, washcloths, pads, linens and any other supplies you will need to clean the patient.
- Generally, if the patient is bed bound, two nurses will be required. Raise the bed to the level that will be comfortable for both nurses. Nurses are notoriously bad at not protecting their backs. Always raise the bed to minimize straining the back. Also, if you have lifts or assistive devices available, use them! If the patient's gown is soiled, go ahead and remove it. Cover the patient with a fresh towel to protect their modesty. First, turn the patient to whichever side is easiest for them. If the patient is able, always ask them to help turn. This helps nurses while increasing patient autonomy and strength.

- If the patient is having loose stool, then you may want to clean their front first and tuck a washcloth or towel between their legs.
- Once the patient is cleaned on the first side, tuck the dirty linen, pad, and wipes under the patient. Try to ensure nothing soiled is touching the patient. Place the fitted sheet on that side and the pad. Roll the new sheet and pad under the soiled linen, again trying to avoid soiling them.
- The patient will now be turned (typically rolled) to the other side. Let the patient know they will roll over a big bump, so they know they know what to anticipate. The second nurse will remove all the soiled items at this point. Then they will clean the patient from the other side, before placing the rest of the fitted sheet and unrolling the rest of the pad.
- If you are giving a complete bed bath, you will generally clean their front before turning them and cleaning their back side.
- The final step is to pull the patient up, if needed, and do any final straightening.

## BOSS TIPS:

- Make sure all lines or tubing are clear prior to turning patients. The last thing you want is for an IV or any other equipment to become dislodged while turning the patient.
- Remove any soiled linen or wipes immediately after finishing. Don't leave poopy linen or trash in the patient's room; this is awful for the patient and anyone else who will come to their room. Spray odor neutralizer if available.

# Chapter 8

............................................................

# I Believe I Can Fly: The Transition to Solo Nurse

I live my life by the philosophy "Don't ask for permission, ask for forgiveness." Unfortunately, my mantra doesn't apply well to nursing. If ever in doubt about ANYTHING (medication, procedure, protocol), ASK someone. Mostly this will be no big deal; someone will clarify for you and you go on your merry way. Sometimes though, a nurse or doctor will act a little huffy and puffy and make you feel incompetent. ASK ANYWAY. You may have a moment when you feel your blood rushing to your ears because you are about to do something and you are not sure if it is right. You don't want to ask because another nurse has already shown you how to do it twice. You are legitimately afraid she is going to bite your head off. We have all been there. ASK ANYWAY. Five minutes of embarrassment will fade away faster than the regret of compromising a patient because you were too scared to ask. If you make a mistake (and we all do), own up to it. Usually the faster a mistake is caught, the faster it can be remedied (if needed) and cause the least amount of harm to the patient.

Another favorite expression of mine is "Fake it till you make it." Unfortunately, this also doesn't apply well to nursing. If you don't know information that a nurse/patient/doctor asks you, don't pretend you do. Incorrect information could result in harm to the patient. Respond with a big smile and say, "Let me find out for you." It's proactive "I don't know-ing." You have in the best way let them know you don't know, but you will try your best to find out.

As you set out to fly solo, let this thought settle in your head: Nursing is not actually a solo sport. The better rapport you can build with your healthcare team, the more successful you will be in providing quality care. Doctors, nurses, respiratory therapists, custodians, secretaries, etc. all play an important role. Don't ever think you are above or below any individual in the healthcare team.

# BOSS TIPS:

- Get friendly with your secretary. She is a genie who will help you find that random doctor's number or document when you have no idea where to look.
- Learn to delegate respectfully and responsibly. We CANNOT do it all. When you need help, delegate the task to someone you can trust and within their scope of practice.
- This one is a personal favorite of mine. Write the most common phone numbers you use on a label and stick it on the back of your badge. These numbers include radiology, lab, pharmacy, blood bank, etc. As a new nurse, it is so handy to have these numbers right on your badge.
- If I were to get a nursing tattoo, it would say CLUSTER CARE. Learn how to group tasks together appropriately to save both time and energy.

Here is a simple example: Let's say a patient has one medication due at 1130 and one at 1200. The patient also has a blood draw scheduled for 1230 (we'll assume you do blood draws on this unit). The novice nurse would go into the room two or three separate times. A boss nurse would give the two medications and bring the blood draw supplies so all three items could be completed in one trip. This not only helps the nurse but helps the patient by minimizing constant interruptions.

## Start of Shift

There is a list of information you will want to know at the start of your shift. Generally you will review the chart while getting report. You may need to spend a few extra minutes after getting report to fill in any gaps. If you are feeling a bit anxious at the start of your nursing career, you can come in 10 minutes early and review this information prior to getting report. If you are not feeling a bit anxious at the start of your nursing career, I would lovingly caution you to "check yo' self before you wreck yo' self." In other words, confidence is sexy, cockiness is not.

## Start of Shift Checklist

- Read patient history and review course of current diagnosis
- Read any doctors' notes for at least the last couple of shifts, specifically progress notes or plan of care notes
- Read through the patient orders and medications
- Read the results of any tests or scans
- Review labs and note trends/abnormalities

Initially this may seem like a lot of information to review, but with practice it will take a matter of minutes.

## Patient Assessment and Nursing Intervention

Or how I like to think of it: What's up with the patient? And what do I do about it?

Being a good nurse isn't about stuffing that poor brain with all medical knowledge. I don't know about you, but my brain isn't anywhere near that big. The clearer and more objective your baseline assessment is, the clearer the appropriate intervention will be when the patient's status changes. The idea is to train your brain to think effectively when faced with the unexpected. Focus on the "big picture," and prioritize critical interventions. Whenever you feel overwhelmed, take a deep breath and ask yourself, "What is the most important action for me to take that will contribute best to the patient's safety and well-being?" The patient's "A-B-C-s" (airway, breathing, and circulation) are always the priority. (Newer ACLS guidelines generally designate circulation, i.e. compressions, to be addressed first in CPR.) ANYTIME a patient's airway, breathing, or circulation is compromised, your immediate intervention will be to correct that compromise. Usually the patient's vitals signs will indicate if there is an acute change in their status. However, be on the lookout for other indicators, such as an acute change in neurological status or lab values. The more familiarity you have for normal findings and normal ranges for lab values, the better your response will be if the patient has a change from baseline. Again, always prioritize the "A-B-Cs", and then progress to less critical interventions.

Let me clarify that I don't go sit in a corner and make a priority list while my patient's vitals are tanking. Assessing, analyzing, and implementing constantly play out in the back of a nurse's head. The more experience you get, the more streamlined this process becomes.

## Time Management and Prioritizing

I approach nursing tasks like a game of "Family Feud." The most important task is at the top of the board, and continues in order of priority. Imagine a board in your mind that is constantly organizing all your tasks in order of most critical importance. Early in your career, it is a great idea to write down these tasks. There are several things you can do to help improve time management.

1. As mentioned before, remember to cluster care as much as possible. For example, if you are going to give a patient their medications at 0900, then ensure you are giving all their medications that are due till 1000. Also, if they have any other interventions that need to be done in the morning, try to gather all necessary supplies and finish those while in the patient's room.

2. Try to organize your shift one hour at a time. When you feel you have too many tasks to finish, focus on all you need to complete in the next hour. At times, thinking about all the tasks that need to be accomplished over the course of a shift feels overwhelming. Take it one hour at a time.

3. Ask for help sooner rather than later. If you feel you are starting to get behind, ask for help before the panic sets in. Some nurses will wait until they are several tasks behind before reaching out for help. If there is someone on the unit who is qualified to help and has the time to, ask them to assist so you don't get too far behind. Remember that some days will be extremely busy, and some days you will be the nurse who has time to help. Be sure to pay it forward to other nurses when you have the time.

Here is a simple tool that can be useful, particularly early in your career. (This tool can be found on kanikaraja.com for your use.)

## Nursing Tasks Shift Breakdown

| | PATIENT 1 MEDS + TASKS | PATIENT 2 MEDS + TASKS | PATIENT 3 MEDS + TASKS | PATIENT 4 MEDS + TASKS |
|---|---|---|---|---|
| 0700-0900 | | | | |
| 0900-1100 | | | | |
| 1100-1300 | | | | |
| 1300-1500 | | | | |
| 1500-1700 | | | | |
| 1700-1900 | | | | |

Time management is a skill that will be developed with practice. Most nurses start to find their time management groove within a year, although some days will be so busy that even 15 years' experience can't keep you from getting behind. When we have multiple interventions that need to be done, we tend to rush and make mistakes that ultimately lead to more time being eaten up. For example, you suddenly remember that your patient had important labs due half an hour ago! You quickly draw them and send them down. In your haste, you put the wrong patient label on the sample. Ultimately, your rush contributed to having to do the task all over again. Mistakes are inevitable in nursing, but stopping to form a plan for a couple minutes can lead to much better time management overall. When that panicky feeling sets in, a two-minute pause button can give your brain the time it needs to reset.

# Chapter 9

## Do Nurses STILL Eat Their Young?

I would say that nurses nowadays are more likely to snack on their young rather than eat them. I forget though, the word "snack" has an entirely different meaning today. I have heard some horrendous stories of both experienced nurses and providers making newer nurses feel completely inadequate, to the point of driving them to quit. The winds are definitely changing though. In my career I have rarely had a nurse or doctor place me under emotional or mental strain. In general, the overall approach of all healthcare providers is much more inclusive and supportive than in the past.

Although, I have had a couple of experiences where the behavior of a fellow nurse has been unreasonably disrespectful. At my first job there was a nurse who seemed to make it a personal mission to cause as much embarrassment to newer nurses as possible. The irony was that this person had only been a nurse herself for about three years. How quickly some forget what it felt like to be a new nurse.

I had a horrible night shift in which I cared for a septic patient who was tanking. First the patient had to be intubated. Then the patient required a central line and arterial line, which the provider put in as fast as possible, as the patient was becoming very hypotensive. I had given several blood products, antibiotics, and started four different vasopressors. (Vasopressors are medications used to constrict blood vessels to increase blood pressure.) I had tried to stabilize the patient all night, and the patient's blood pressure was finally at an acceptable level at approximately 0630. Lo and behold, I was giving report to my favorite nurse!

"Stacey" had an orientee with her that day and I gave them both report. Stacey asked me a couple of questions, which I could tell she was assuming I wouldn't know the answer to, but I was on it like orange on a pumpkin. I was just about to leave feeling quite content with myself when Stacey, in her saccharine sweet tone, said, "Kanika, can you come here for a minute?" My mind began beating an angry drum. I did everything I could, now what is her problem?! I went back into the patient's room and she spoke directly to her orientee (Stacey did not face me or make eye contact with me). She told the orientee, "This central line dressing is bloody and not labeled. You want to make sure you are not this kind of nurse when you are off orientation." I stared in disbelief and a barrage of silent F-bombs were catapulting in my brain. It had been one of the most difficult shifts I'd had since being off orientation, and I left work feeling completely defeated. Yes, it is best practice to make sure all dressings are clean and labeled, but to focus on that one detail considering the shift I had was spiteful. I should have addressed the situation at the time, but just left with my blood boiling. I am generally good at letting things go, but my frustration towards her still remains to this day.

I had a similar incident not too long ago, but I no longer tolerate that kind of nonsense. I had a provider (neither a doctor or nurse actually) who was condescending and rude in her interactions with me. I let it slide once, but the second time I walked up to her and simply said, "It seems like you have some kind of problem with me. If you could tell me what it is, then we can fix it and move on." She looked surprised and huffily said, "It's nothing." I flashed a huge smile and responded, "Ok, then." I had addressed her face-to-face in a calm manner, and there was nothing left for me to stress or get upset about.

As I said before, my list of negative instances is a short one. The list of times when I was drowning and my fellow nurses came to the rescue is a much longer one. Whenever you interact with a person who treats you disrespectfully, don't let them become your Stacey. Address the issue calmly and immediately so you can be rid of the nagging feeling that you should say something. The worst offense of them all would be to become a Stacey. You can address any issue without being an *sshole. Don't eat or snack on anybody; they have cookies for that, y'all.

# Chapter 10

## Rapids and Crash Carts and Codes, Oh My!

My nursing buddy and I saw the flatline on the monitor at the same time. We swiveled to face each other for a split second and then he ran into the room. I was a couple steps behind him and he had just placed his hands on the patient's chest, prepared to do compressions. I yelled out, "He's a DNR (Do Not Resuscitate)!" My friend had just done one compression in a rush of adrenaline before he registered what I had said. He looked sheepishly at me and said, "I only did one." I desperately checked for a pulse and found absolutely nothing. As I stared down at the patient, a solitary thought kept hammering in my head: "You told his wife to go home and get some rest." You told his wife to go home and get some rest. You told his wife to go home and get some rest!" I felt eons go by, but in reality, about 19 seconds went by. Suddenly, the patient opened his eyes and was startled to find us on either side of him. I gasped, "How do you feel, sir?" He grinned and said, "Like I just took the world's best nap!" My fellow nurse still maintains that that one compression was like hitting the reset button, and that is what brought the patient back bright-eyed and smiling!

The first time a patient of yours goes into cardiopulmonary arrest (which will generally be referred to as a code blue), it will cause an adrenaline rush unlike anything you have ever felt before. However, the longer you work in intensive care, the more familiar the rhythm of a code will become. There is an Advanced Cardiac Life Support (ACLS) algorithm, which is not overly complex once you become familiar with it. The patient that suddenly loses a pulse and stops breathing will always be scary, but your skill during a code will become refined over time, similar to any other skill. If you decide to work in an adult intensive care unit, then an ACLS class will be mandatory. However, all acute care nurses can benefit from both an ECG and ACLS class. It is helpful to understand what factors might lead to a patient going into cardiac arrest, so early signs of deterioration can be detected, especially if the patient is not in ICU. This is where a Code Rapid Response and a Rapid Response Team will come into play.

I will clarify several terms before we move on:

Code Rapid Response: An alert that is called to intervene when a patient (not in Intensive Care) is deteriorating suddenly, usually in an attempt to avoid the patient having a cardiac or respiratory arrest.

Rapid Response Team: A team of designated healthcare professionals that responds to a rapid response. Most hospitals will have a protocol on how to initiate a rapid, and what conditions may warrant a rapid being called.

A few examples of conditions that may trigger a Rapid Response:

- an acute change in the vital signs
- an acute change in the patient's level of consciousness
- any significant bleeding from an operative site, chest tube, etc.

Remember that a rapid response relies greatly on nursing intuition. If you are concerned about a patient's condition but unsure whether a rapid response is necessary, ask your charge nurse or even a rapid response team member. Trust the gut! If your gut strongly tells you something is wrong, trust it and act accordingly.

Code Blue: An emergency event where a patient is in cardiopulmonary arrest. Usually, a hospital-wide alert is sent and the appropriate healthcare providers respond.

Crash Cart: a wheeled container that has life-saving equipment (including a defibrillator) and medications typically used during a code blue.

Make sure you learn your unit's protocol on how to initiate a Rapid and/or Code Blue. Also, become familiar with the crash cart. Know where it is located on your unit, and have basic knowledge about which items are stored in which drawers. Have your preceptor also review use of the unit-specific defibrillator with you.

Although the algorithm of ACLS will be taught in the specific ACLS class, I want to give you several tips on how to become more comfortable during a code situation.

## BOSS TIPS:

- Try to respond to as many codes as you can while in orientation. However, if there is no clear way for you to be helpful during a code, then it may be better to step out. The ultimate goal of code is to be as streamlined as possible, and often there are way too many people hanging out in the room without serving any purpose. Don't be someone who adds to the chaos. I think I hear a faint "AMEN!" from all ICU nurses in the distance.

- During your first couple of codes, the only role you may be comfortable with is giving compressions. You will still learn a lot about the flow of a code, even while being in this role.

- Fill a variety of roles as your comfort level grows. These roles include recorder, giving medications, and manning the defibrillator. If the team leader assigns you a role, then verbalize that you understand and will assume the role.

- In the event the team leader assigns you a role that you feel unsafe or uncomfortable performing, make it clear to them so the role can be reassigned. If you see a role that needs to be filled, then verbalize that you will be taking that role.

- If it is your patient that codes, start thinking (though the primary focus is on performing the action of the code) about reversible causes and about what questions the provider will likely ask. These questions might include admitting diagnosis, relevant history, most recent labs, allergies, and cardiac history.

- Always loudly vocalize that you understood any order from a provider and when the order is being carried out. For example, if the provider asks you to draw up 1mg of epinephrine and administer it, verbalize "Drawing up 1mg of epinephrine. 1mg of epinephrine given and flushed in." Try to always speak clearly and in the direction of the team leader/provider who gave the order.

## Code Status and Advocating for the Patient

In my story at the start of the chapter, my patient had elected to have a DNR (Do Not Resuscitate) status. In rarer cases, a patient may designate a DNI (Do Not Intubate) status or may designate they do not want CPR performed if they have a cardiac arrest. Whatever code status your patient chooses, ensure it is clearly designated in the patient's electronic and paper chart.

It is our duty to respect our patient's wishes in regard to their end-of-life care and life-saving efforts. If a patient's wishes do not correlate with their code status, then be an advocate for them and facilitate a discussion with the healthcare team and the patient's family. People often ask me if constantly dealing with death is overwhelmingly sad. As sad as death can be, there is a scenario far more painful. When a patient is kept alive past the point where they will have meaningful life left, it weighs far heavier than the pain of death. Despite the most well-intentioned advice from the healthcare team, some patient's families will elect to have every intervention done until the last beat and breath. However, let your nursing heart be light with the knowledge that you have done all that you could to advocate for the patient.

# Chapter 11

## Night of the Living Dead, AKA Night Shift

I was working a one-and-done night shift, which is my term for when I am working for just one night. Now that I have explained what a one-and-done night shift is, I realize that it really didn't need much explanation. Anyhoo.

I had plans to meet up with a non-nursey friend for breakfast the next morning. I had a relatively good night with no major issues. I left the hospital feeling at peace with the world and coated my lips with my cherry-hued chapstick, dabbed more of the same on my cheeks and thought I didn't look half bad. I met my friend at the cafe and the first words out of her mouth were, "Oh my god Kanika, was last night awful?" I responded, "Actually it wasn't too bad, why do you think that?" She looked a little embarrassed and said, "Oh nothing." I prodded her further and it finally escaped her lips, "It's just that you look half dead." Suffice it to say we are no longer friends. Alright, we are friends, because she was right and she is a wonderful person whose filter just needs to be changed more often.

I worked the night shift for four years before I made the transition to day shift. I am naturally a morning person, and unless I am dancing or gabbing, my eyelids are fighting by 11 p.m. I was reluctant to go to day shift as the thought of occupational therapy, physical therapy, speech therapy, and social work, and doctors, and family, and lord knows who else would completely overwhelm me. Also, I once worked a day shift on the Medical Surgical Unit (I was floated from ICU) and the morning medication administration took me until about 11 a.m. I had both discharges and admissions throughout the shift. On top of everything else, my night shift self forgot I had to actually give the patients meal trays on day shift! Because, you know, people eat and stuff like that during the daytime. That one shift deterred me from day shift for another year, but I recently took a deep breath and made the leap! Day shift can be daunting, but my body and mind thank me everyday for making the switch.

Even though I have been throwing around the "day shift is awesome" confetti, night shift also has its perks.

## Perks of working nights

• No getting up early

Some people do not jive with early morning starts. If the thought of waking at 5 a.m. makes you want to curl up into the fetal position, night shift may be a great option for you.

• Slower pace

Oftentimes, new grads will start out on night shift and it can be beneficial to start off there. Generally, night shift has a slower pace and a lack of ancillary staff (ie. PT, OT, case management).

This allows the nurse to get to know the patient more in depth as, most of the time, the only person the patient interacts with is the nurse.

- Greater autonomy
Even though I said that there is a slower pace at night, there are many exceptions. Sometimes night shift can be extremely busy as there is much less support staff at night time. The reduced staff may mean the nurse has to become more self-reliant in terms of problem solving. For example, during a code on night shift, there may not be as much staff, therefore it will fall on the nurses to assume greater responsibility.

- Increased pay
Generally, night shifters have the added benefit of a slight pay boost. Shift differential will vary from facility to facility, but the hourly rate can be $2-$5 more on night shift. Cha-ching!

- Camaraderie
This one is more of a personal observation. Since there is less staff and family around at night, night shift staff seem to develop a unique and weird bond. I have had some deep and strange conversations with fellow nurses at 3 a.m., and have shared things that I have never shared with a fellow day shift nurse. If you have worked nights, you know exactly what I am talking about.

We have established that there are benefits to working nights, but how can you make your body adjust to the "graveyard" shift? For those of you who are naturally night owls, this may not be so difficult. However, if you are like me, you may need a little help making it through the night. I am going to provide you with my top tips. Warning: I am going to include tips such as: limit caffeine intake. I can collectively hear y'all thinking, "Kanika be crazy" at the thought of limiting caffeine on a 12-hour night shift.

To begin with, I am going to describe my ideal sleep schedule while I was working night shift. I reiterate: you will find your own groove for the sleeping pattern on night shift, as you will find your groove for everything in nursing. But as you are finding your ideal mix, mine can provide you a foundation which you can build on.

## One-shift sleeping pattern

If I am only working one night shift (7 p.m. to 7 a.m.) before I have a night off, I wake up around 8 a.m., stay up till around 1 p.m., and then sleep until 4 to 5 p.m. depending on what I need to do before I go into work. The next morning when I get off, I go to bed by 10 a.m. and wake up between 2 to 3 p.m. There are many nurses who will power through the day on their last night working and go to bed directly that night after 9 p.m. I have NEVER been able to pull that off. After a 12-hour night shift, I will always require a solid 4 to 5 hours of sleep before I become something resembling a human again. When you start on night shift, I would advise you to get adequate rest before and after your shift. If you find that you are one of these "vampire" nurses who seem to survive well on less sleep, then more power to you. However, initially be cautious and make sure your body doesn't break down from lack of sleep.

## BOSS TIP:

If you find that you are becoming sick easily when you first start night shift, the simple answer may be staring you straight in the face. Get more sleep!

## Multiple-shift sleeping pattern

If I am working multiple nights shifts in a row, I again wake up around 8 a.m. the day of my first shift, sleep at 1 p.m., and then up by around 4 to 5 p.m. The next day after I get off of work, I would go to bed again by 10 a.m. and sleep till 4 to 5 p.m. I would keep repeating this same pattern until I am not working another night, and again on my last night I would sleep in until 2 to 3 p.m. the next day.

## Other night shift tips

- When I started working night shift, a nurse told me to eat breakfast foods before I came into work to trick my body into thinking it was daytime. Since breakfast food is amazing, I gave it a shot. In fact, one of the most amazing TV characters of all time said, "Why would anybody ever eat anything besides breakfast food?" To which the other brilliant character responded, "People are idiots, Leslie." If you know where this reference is from, then I already know I like you. I followed the breakfast advice for the first few months and found it helpful. Also, since eggs are pretty much the world's easiest food to make and give a nice little boost of protein, they can be a nice pre-work meal.
- Get your caffeine in early. I would stay away from a triple-shot latte anytime after 1 a.m. Some night shift nurses are immune to caffeine (or so they think), and having caffeine later in the shift doesn't affect their sleep pattern. However, if you have any trouble sleeping after the night shift, then you want your last several hours of the shift to be caffeine-free so you can catch some zzzs when the shift is over. I also limit myself to one coffee a night because

any more than that and I start feeling jittery. Also, when I increase my caffeine intake but then try to stop or reduce, I get headaches. So I find that one cup is the magic number for me!

- Snacks on snacks on snacks

    I am a HUGE snacker. Any chip, cookie, or cracker better dodge my grubby little hands to remain safe from my hunger. Luckily, I enjoy healthy food and snacks just as much as unhealthy ones. To avoid gorging on foods with high sugar or high sodium, which make me feel like dancing for 12 minutes and then leave me slumped over in my chair afterwards, I ensure that my lunch bag is brimming with healthy(ish) snacks. Some of my favorites include:

    - hummus/guacamole with pita or carrot sticks
    - nuts (flavored almonds and walnuts are my fave)
    - Greek yogurt
    - fruit (grapes and berries are my choice) and cheese
    - peanut or almond butter
    - popcorn
    - oatmeal
    - dark chocolate

- Water for the win

    I find the simplest way to get myself to drink enough water is to bring a water bottle, bonus points if I doctor it up with some natural flavor. My favorite add-ins include lemon juice, raspberries, mint, orange, pineapple, and basil (a bit weird but quite tasty). Also, if I find that my shift is going slowly, I drink more water throughout the shift to let my bathroom trips keep me awake. Since my bladder is the size of a large walnut, this can be an effective method for staying awake. Be cautious you don't go crazy with this tip, I don't want to cause any electrolyte imbalances, y'all! Staying hydrated really helps to minimize the sluggishness that night shift can cause.

- Staying Awake — the lesser-known Bee Gees hit

  Some nights will be so busy that your butt and your chair will remain strangers and never get to meet (AKA you will never sit down. The best jokes are the ones that have to be explained!). However, when you have a slow night, stay active. Walk around the unit and see if anyone needs help. One of my favorite and funniest nurses I knew would do lunges up and down the hall to keep from getting sleepy. Call her crazy, but come springtime she was bikini ready! Some nurses do well with a cat nap during their break on night shift, but I always find that I feel extra groggy and cranky post nap.

- Sleeping in the daytime

  Luckily I can pretty much sleep on cue. Seriously, you can have a mariachi band playing in the background and it will not disturb my sleep. However, I know some nurses struggle with sleeping during the day. Some of the remedies that I have heard help include:
  - Blackout curtains
  - White noise machines
  - Keeping your bedroom at a cool temperature

- My Kryptonite — the drive back home

  The absolute worst part of working night shift is the drive back home. If it is cold outside and I have to turn the heater on, forget about it. A warm car and an exhausted body is a horrible combination. Every cell in my body will gently whisper, "Let's just close those eyes for a few minutes." One factor for my decision to switch to day shift was I felt less and less safe driving home. I do think I fall on the extreme end of the spectrum, and hopefully your body doesn't respond as poorly on the drive back home. However, please be cautious and do pull over if you find the fatigue is getting to an unsafe level. There are several techniques I utilized on drives home that may be helpful to you as well.

- Carpool/Call someone

On a couple of my travel assignments, I was lucky enough to make friends who lived close enough to me that we carpooled on nights we were both working. Not only does the company help to keep from getting sleepy, but it can become a pseudo therapy session. It felt great to be able to vent any frustrations or just joke about crazy events from the shift before. If carpooling with someone for some of your shifts is an option, I highly recommend it. If carpooling is not an option, then call someone who can chat with you on your way home. This is the perfect time to catch up with your mom and hear her complain about how complicated her new cell phone is.

- Embrace the cold

On cold days when I was feeling extra sleepy, I would keep my window cracked. The sharp stream of air on my face would sometimes be just the slap I needed to keep myself alert. As I mentioned before, I wouldn't allow myself the luxury of keeping the car too warm because that would buy me a one-way ticket to passing out.

- Turn on the tunes

It blows my mind how amazing a singer I am in my car when no one else is listening. Does anyone else have the same problem? Then for some reason, when I hear my voice on a recording, I sound like a cow in labor. The cow just sent in a statement which reads, "Nope, don't put me in the same boat as you, girl." Anyway, my favorite method of staying sharp on the way home is turning my car into a concert and belting my heart out.

- Ridesharing/public transport
  When I did a travel assignment in LA, I chose not to bring my car to avoid parking hassles. Since I lived only a couple of miles away from the hospital, using Lyft and Uber was a convenient and economical option. When I did a travel assignment close to San Francisco, I was able to use a metro line that brought me within a five-minute walk to work. I truly enjoyed not utilizing a car in both of those cities, as parking can be ridiculously difficult and driving can be tedious. Both ridesharing and public transport kept me from worrying about driving and gave me a feel of the local vibe and culture. I only made the stereotypical mistake once. Once on my train ride home in SF, I fell asleep and woke up approximately an hour from home!

## My farewell love letter to night shift

I made the switch to day shift only six months ago, so if you will give me just a moment, I want to write night shift a little farewell note.

Dear night shift,

I want to thank you for all that you have taught me. You have allowed me to get to know my patients in depth, both their medical history and their personal story. You have made me understand the value of teamwork, and because of you I have met some wonderful weirdo nurses. I have developed a twisted sense of humor because of you, and I owe my ability to eat and sleep on cue all to you. I used to be a cranky napper, and now I nap like a boss.

Night shift, treat the next generation of nurses with tender, loving care. Give them enough energy to not require six shots of espresso per shift, let them sleep like logs during the daytime, and please don't let the attending doctor yell at them when they call for an order at 3 a.m.

Though the time came for us to part ways, I am sending you a truly bad'ss group of nurses to take my place. I wish you all the best, and will remember you fondly. However, the time has come for me to say, "Thank you, next."

Yours truly, Kanika

P.S. I blame you for my gray hairs.

# Chapter 12

## When It Gets Too Hard

I sat in the car after my second clinical shift and my hands were visibly trembling. The tears that had fought so hard all day finally lost the battle. I cried a big, sloppy, ugly cry and I genuinely thought F this. My heart isn't strong enough for me to be a nurse.

The day had started off the same as any other clinical day. I was assigned a nurse to shadow on a medical surgical floor. We were making our initial rounds and introducing ourselves to the assigned patients. One of our patients had been admitted for urgent dialysis. She also had an extensive medical history and had been brought in via ambulance. A neighbor of hers had become concerned when he didn't see her for several days and had called the police, who found her in her house. She was a dialysis patient who had missed several treatments and was admitted to the hospital. One of her many other conditions was severe plaque psoriasis.

The memory of walking into her room and meeting her is permanently etched into my mind. Her entire body was covered with what appeared to look like thick, crusty scales. She had a slight build and was soft spoken. She was withdrawn and answered in mostly one- or two-word responses. I remember that her eyes looked sunken and she had the body language of someone who was used to so much pain that she was simply alive and no longer truly living.

A wound care nurse had been assigned to her to address her severe plaque psoriasis. The wound care nurse was seeing her the day of my clinical. She asked if I would like to assist the patient in her treatment. Her treatment consisted of her receiving a whirl-pool bath to slough off the outer layer (essentially the "scaly" layer) of the skin and the application of the prescribed ointment. To be honest, the sight and smell of the psoriasis (her skin had areas that were oozing) was making my stomach turn. I felt guilty about feeling this way and told myself, "Come on Kanika, you have to get used to seeing such conditions as a nurse. Of course you can power through this."

I apologize in advance as the next part is graphic, but I am only including the details for you to get an understanding of what I was feeling. We wheeled the patient to the therapy room and helped her to get into the whirlpool tub. As the water swirled around her body, slowly the top layer of her skin began sloughing off. Her freshly exposed skin under the plaques was raw, red and looked... angry. The whole time while in the bath, she was gently grimacing, but again in the deflected way of someone who is too used to this pain. At this point, the wound care nurse told me, "The bath has several more minutes left, I am going to grab a towel from the linen cart. Be right back!"

I felt anxious about being left with the patient and felt that I needed to cut the silence by engaging the patient in casual conversation. Unfortunately, when I am nervous in any situation, I don't do well with quiet. I feel a need to fill it with my nervous chatter.

I asked a couple of questions while being completely aware that I should probably stop talking and leave the lady in peace. She answered my questions distractedly, without really looking towards me. As I opened my mouth to ask yet another question, the patient suddenly grabbed my hand and looked directly into my eyes. She said with conviction, "Please sweetie, can't y'all just let me die? I am so tired of living. I don't have any family to live for. I don't see the point of doing all this when I have nothing to live for."

I stared back at the patient, and my mouth opened and closed several times as I struggled to find an appropriate response to what I had just heard. The wound care nurse came back several moments later, and the patient turned away from me and again gazed quietly into the distance. I was stunned by the patient's words, and the rest of the day passed in a haze. To this day I cannot remember if I properly expressed to her assigned nurse about how hopeless the patient felt or asked about palliative care. I would love to believe that I intervened in some meaningful way, but if I am being honest, I don't think I did. I still wonder if the patient had made anyone else aware of her feelings, or had only conveyed them to me the one time. My reaction to a similar situation would be completely different now. I would have asked the patient to elaborate and tried to understand what needed to be done to improve the situation. I would have immediately notified the physician and asked about palliative care, social work, and a more in-depth psychiatric evaluation.

As I said before, nursing has a steep learning curve. There is a learning curve not only with nursing knowledge but also with how to manage the emotional aspect of the job. Over time my knowledge, skill, and ability to respond to difficult situations have grown. I can't tell you the last time my job has made me cry. My nursing heart hasn't become hard or calloused, but it has grown stronger.

I don't care any less for my patients than when I started nursing, but my heart recognizes that carrying a burden doesn't lighten the patient's load. I try to focus all my energy on action on their behalf, and have accepted that I can't solve every problem.

Whenever I feel overwhelmed, I always come back to one simple thought: "I am here to reduce fear." I think hospitals can be terrifying, and if I can care for someone in a way that reduces their fear and pain, then I can't think of anything else I'd rather do. Rather than letting emotions drown me, I focus on my one little mantra. Although fixing bodies is what I do, it is not why I do it. Anytime I have a crappy day at work and am running in circles, I take a deep breath and remember why I choose to do this. "I am here to reduce fear." Whenever it gets too hard, do two things: ask for help, and come back to one simple thought of why you do this. You got this.

# Chapter 13

## Take Care You

Nursing is hard. Thank you for that revolutionary insight, Kanika. What other revelations do you have for us? Puppies are cute? The sun is hot? Yes, it goes without saying that nursing is a difficult line of work, the most essential aspects of which I have tried to cover in this book. I want you to do something right now. What I am about to ask you to do is weird, but you are a nurse (or about to become one), and weird is right up our alley. Say out loud right now, "I WILL take care of myself." If you are in an airplane or in a coffee shop reading this book, all the better. Having people perceive you as slightly off can totally work in your favor. I guarantee if you are on a plane and you loudly say, "I will take care of myself," the person next to you is definitely going to give you a little more elbow room, and if there is an open seat close by, they may even move! Alright, jokes aside, make a commitment to your own well-being.

No nursing unit will be ideal, and you may find your patient load to be overwhelming. This is pretty normal for nursing. However, do a mental check every few months to assess if anything within reasonable reach can be changed to make you happier and healthier. Sometimes, the best thing you can do is to remind yourself, "It's okay to not be okay". Many hospitals have resources, (such as counseling), to help with the emotional aspect of the job. You could also speak to a manager, colleague, or friend. Reaching out to someone doesn't mean you are not strong. All it means is, you are smart enough to ask for a little help.

There are two questions I suggest asking yourself as part of your self-care process. If the answer to either of these questions is consistently a no, then form a plan to improve the situation.

1) Do I feel supported at my current job?

It is no secret that nursing units are often understaffed for a variety of reasons. The amount of work isn't quite as important as your work environment. Do you work with coworkers who have your back? Does management take your feedback into consideration? Managers absolutely do not have the power to solve every problem, but the good ones will take feedback, especially when there is a similar concern from several employees, and try to form some sort of solution. Do I have opportunities for growth and education? I would give any job a solid year before forming an absolute opinion, but after one year if you are miserable going to work, it may be time to consider a new position.

2) Do I feel healthy?

Let's delve a little deeper into this question. Ask yourself if you are physically, mentally, and emotionally tuning up as needed. It is insane how we often take better care of our cars and gutters than ourselves. One aspect of nursing (and life) that I have had to grapple with is being vocal when I am not feeling healthy or happy. It has taken me a long time to realize that vulnerability isn't weakness.

It takes the most courage to face an issue head on and only then can a solution be found.

## A Quick Note on Body Mechanics

Use good ones. For the love of all that is good and pure in this world, raise that bed to the appropriate height before turning and repositioning your patient. If you are asking, "Kanika, have you always used proper body mechanics?" Of course I have! That hunch I have in my back has always been there.

## Take Care Kanika

Of course, all of us will have different activities that will calm the crazies inside and get us back to feeling good again. I am providing a few of my own (keepin' it PG y'all) that you are welcome to steal or serve as a springboard to form your own self care plan.

## Yoga:

During my first assignment as a travel nurse, I found a hot yoga studio about two minutes from my apartment. I had never been to a hot yoga class and let me tell you, after the "I'm going to pass out feeling" passed, I was in heaven. A good yoga session (hot or not) fits me as well as sunshine fits the beach. I always feel a lovely combination of strength and relaxation after a class.

## The Outdoors:

I am a bit of a wild child at heart. I feel most at home outside, and my least favorite thing about nursing is that it has to take place indoors. 'Cause of infection control or whatever. On my days off, you will usually find me hiking, playing tennis, or in the nearest water body. Being in nature (or at least outside) helps keep my stir-crazy tendencies at bay.

## Water:

I do try my best to eat a well-balanced diet that includes a lot of veggies, fruits, and cake. I said it was balanced, not perfect. If all else fails in my diet and I have one of those "cereal for dinner" weeks, then I at least drink eight glasses of water a day. Drinking enough water is a club that you probably have been beaten over the head with, but trust me, your skin and body will thank you for it.

## Side Hustle:

Another aspect of nursing that is tricky for me is the lack of creative outlet. I can't draw. I love to sing, but singing doesn't love me. I love to dance, and ok, I'll admit dancing and I have a bit of a fling going. However, I have found that my best outlet has become writing. The inception of this book began exactly there. I wanted a creative endeavor that could also aid others. And BAM! This book was born.

## Non-Nursing:

If you call the IT department, they are likely to ask you if you have tried turning the computer off and on again. (A little wink to another amazing tv show) Sometimes the only thing needed is a simple reboot, and the kinks are magically worked out on their own. Similarly, the best way to refresh the nursing program in your brain is simply by turning it off. This advice is coming from the nurse who in her spare time is writing a book on nursing. Rich. However, believe me when I tell you that I have become really good at shutting my nursing switch off when I am not either in the hospital or writing.

# BOSS TIP:

I want to reinforce something I said early on in the book. Take your first year as a nurse, suck out all the skills and knowledge you have acquired and toss the rest in the garbage. This tip is for anyone who after their first year feels like, "Fuuuuuudge. What have I gotten myself into?" This was me. I did not like being a nurse my first year and wasn't sure whether that feeling was going to change. I am happy to say that it has. My first year, I chose to marinate in my fear and it made me a little too tender. It is an ideal scenario for a chicken, not so ideal for this chick. I am tougher now. I am honored to do my job, and most days it's pretty fun, too.

# Chapter 14

......................................................

# Where Can Nursing Take Me?

When I imagined how I wanted this book to read, a video game hack guide is what always came to mind. I have told you the nursing version of where the crocodiles are, where the quicksand is, and how to get that stash of gold coins. I have focused on how to avoid the traps or simply blast through them. If we have established nothing else in this book, it is that nursing is freakin' hard, yo. Now it is time to focus on the exact opposite. Let's talk about the fact that you have already made the most boss decision of all by choosing to become a nurse.

I have heard the phrase, "The possibilities are endless" in regards to decisions where there are about three options. This expression was made for nursing, where the options truly feel endless. You can work at a clinic, hospital, school, private company, etc. You can work in pediatrics, geriatrics, psychiatry, surgery, delivery, emergency, etc. You can make a solid income as a new graduate with a bachelor's; actually, it is one of the highest starting salaries for a bachelor's degree. You can progress by getting your master's, and potentially your doctorate. You can work in administration, education, or as a more traditional practitioner. Your path and options are limited only by your imagination.

I haven't even mentioned my favorite part of nursing yet: TRAVEL. Travel nursing was an absolute game changer for me. I literally broke out into a jig when I realized that I had chosen a profession that would pay me to travel almost anywhere in the U.S. for three-month assignments. Let's go on a little journey, shall we? Let's begin by surfing in Hawaii, skiing in Colorado, catching a Broadway show in New York, and wrap it up by listening to jazz while eating beignets in Louisiana. Not only that, the salary that most travelers make allows them to take periods of time off between assignments to pursue other passions.

There was a brief period of time in my life where I toyed with the idea of becoming a doctor. The brief period passed like a fart in the wind, or something poetic like that. I thank the heavens every day that I did not pursue this option. While it is a brilliant path for some, it was not the right choice for me. The thought of eight years in medical school still gives me more goosebumps than "The Conjuring." This leads me to another aspect that I love about this job. In every position that I have held, I have rarely had to be on call or work after hours. I try to give the best of myself when I am working my 12 hours. However, once I clock out, I am delighted by the knowledge that my time is truly my time. I don't carry home presentations that need to be worked on, or have to do international conference calls, or do much planning for the next day. Nurses often have the option of working one or two shifts a week, instead of the usual three. Even the inception of this book was allowed by the fact that for one of my contracts, I gave myself the luxury of only working two days a week instead of three.

Take a moment to digest a beautiful truth. You are about to become a superhero. Yes, you will get pooped on and yelled at. However, you will directly make an impact on hundreds of lives and become the boss storyteller in your group of friends.

No disrespect to the accountants out there, but what is their version of a crazy day? A day when a spreadsheet is missing a column, so every item is off by one? You will have stories that will literally cause soda to shoot out of your friend's nose.

I feel a little bit like a mother hen who has just hatched all her chickies and now all that is left is to let them out of the coop. Or maybe that metaphor is too much? I don't need y'all calling human resources telling them that the crazy book lady is talking about sitting on you. Let's see if we can end this on a less weird note. I want to wish each of you the best for your nursing careers. I am not gently wafting positive vibes your way; I am aggressively catapulting them at you. May you always be confident in your skill and knowledge, but never stop learning. May you bite that tongue hard when you are about to be condescending to a patient or colleague. May you never take sh*t from anyone, because ain't nobody got time for that, especially since we will literally be taking sh*t from people. May you feel fulfilled and proud of the difference you make.

The second time you read this book, turn it into a fun little game. Do a squat every time you read the word nurse or nursing. Your booty will be looking like J-Lo by the time you are done.

Made in the USA
Columbia, SC
11 September 2020

18840541R00065